Boy

Anna Hamilton

Between the Lines
PUBLISHING
"An Indie for Indies"

Liminal Books is an imprint of Between the Lines Publishing. The Liminal Books name and logo are trademarks of Between the Lines Publishing.

Copyright © 2021 by Anna Hamilton

Cover design by Suzanne Johnson

Between the Lines Publishing
410 Caribou Trail
Lutsen, MN 55612
btwnthelines.com

First Published: May 2021

ISBN: (Paperback) 978-1-950502-40-0
ISBN: (Ebook) 978-1-950502-41-7

Library of Congress Control Number: 2021937927

Boy

Boy is dedicated to my clan, the Hamilton's. Without them, there would be no me.

I would also like to dedicate this story to all of the people I used as characters in Boy. Although your character is not true to who you are, you are very real and a patch on the quilt of my life. Thank you.

My name is Boy. It's a name that was given to me by Old Man's wife. Old Man is the one who found me. Wife is the one who saved me.

I have no memory before that day—the day I woke up on my back, lying in a pile of leaves in someone's yard, afraid and unable to move. I had no idea where I was or how I got there, but I remember feeling relieved that I wasn't on my stomach. To be face down, with only a view of the dirt and all that crawls within it, would've been my doom for sure.

Above was a canopy of massive tree limbs—slivers of an aqua sky peeking through the woven branches, shielding me from the direct sun, yet allowing me warmth and a view. I'd guessed that it must be October, possibly even November, because I could smell the rot and decay of a summer's growth. A cool breeze brought with it the scent of naked fields after a harvest, confirming the time of year. How I knew this, I didn't know for sure, but the knowledge calmed me enough so that I began to watch the squirrels run around through the brown leaves, scavenging acorns and anything else worthy of stashing for the coming winter. They ran up and down the trunk of an old tree, back and forth along the branches they went. I was relieved that they paid no attention to me.

Fragments of rope poked through the bark of one of the tree limbs, suggesting a long-abandoned swing once hung there—a remnant of another time. To my left was a small white house with faded yellow shutters. Flower boxes hung below the windows, empty and rotting, falling away from themselves

1

board by board, pieces broken and splintered on the ground near where I lay.

To my right, I could see the side of a barn and the rooftops of other small buildings tucked in alongside it. I struggled to see more, but the pain in my head forced me to stop. Exhausted, I closed my eyes and—oddly enough—I fell asleep. The slam of a door shook me awake, and instantly I was reminded of how vulnerable I was. I tried to turn my head towards the sound, but the pain limited my ability to move anything but my eyes.

I was petrified when I saw an old man and the shell of a woman walking in my direction, their footsteps growing louder as they shuffled through the dry leaves. I closed my eyes and held my breath, hoping I would be invisible, terrified that the next crunch would be me. When the crunching stopped, so did the warmth of the sun. A chill ran up my spine when I realized that they hovered over me, casting me in shadow.

I opened my eyes just wide enough to take a peek, and sure enough, there was the old man. He bent a little closer to me, the wrinkles on his face fell forward, exposing sad, investigating eyes.

I blinked once, maybe twice, and then he blinked back at me. as he straightened his crooked body, he said, "Wife, take a look at this little guy. He must be what hit our window this morning."

At least now I had a clue as to why I lay in this yard, unable to move. I closed my eyes again, only tighter this time, hoping they would both just disappear. But when they didn't,

I thought I might as well face my fate. If death was coming, I sure didn't want to miss it. So, I opened my eyes and simply watched them watch me.

The old man waited but received no reply from the one he called "Wife." She was an itty-bitty thing with short gray hair and a blank stare dulling her hooded topaz eyes. Her flowered dress was stained with what looked like food, and not necessarily recent food.

She was close enough to me that I could smell urine. The stench was strong and fresh, not old like the food painting her dress.

Tightening his arm around her small frame, the old man tried to steer her away, back through the yard to the house with the faded shutters. She mumbled something and shook her head in refusal, moving away from him and planting her feet inches from where I lay. Another step and I would be flat as a pancake.

Tears filled the old man's eyes as he pleaded with her to return to the house for a hot cup of tea. But she ignored him, pointing at me, and attempting to bend down. Old Man grabbed hold of her like his life depended on it, but I guessed it was more her life than his. Maybe both, who knows?

I looked away from the eyes that bore into me. I looked to the sky and then to the tree, frantically searching for the squirrels. I searched for anything but Wife because Death is all I saw in her.

Still pointing, she whispered, "Boy."

Old Man cleared his throat. "What?" he asked. "What did you say?" He leaned in and put his face close to hers, hoping for more, as a gust of wind swooped in from across the fields, claiming the loose leaves from the ground and taking with it some of the thick emptiness that surrounded the two of them.

The power of the wind nearly knocked the old woman over, despite the strong arm still clutching her little waist. Like an anchor in a storm, he held on, and once the wind subsided, Old Man gently straightened their bodies. As he did, Wife turned and faced him. "Boy," she repeated firmly.

Something sparkled behind her eyes. I saw it, and I think Old Man saw it too, because a grin spread across his face as he finally succeeded in steering her around towards the house and away from me.

My heart was pounding so hard that I looked down at my chest, fully expecting it to explode right there and then. When it didn't, I stole a glance in their direction, watching the two crooked bodies shuffle through the leaves and into the little house.

Once they were gone, the autumn sun shone down on me again, warming my aching bones. I was safe for the moment, though physically exhausted from fear. At last, I fell asleep again.

OLD MAN AND WIFE

Hugh sat his wife down in a worn, wooden chair—one of the six that he made so long ago for his new bride and anticipated family. The chairs matched the carved oak table, once glowing and clean, now dusty and scattered with crumbs and stacks of paper.

It was at this table that for sixty-one years they had their meals. It was there they enjoyed their family and friends. They laughed and cried at this table. It was the morning meeting place for the farm hands as they discussed the chores ahead. It was where their son Charly did his homework and spit out his peas during supper when no one was looking.

Now it is simply a resting spot for Hugh and Betty. The friends are gone, most of them dead like their families. There is no longer chatter or laughter or Betty's delicious home cooked meals. The farm is no longer worked by the family, but now is leased out. They'd gotten rid of all the animals when Betty fell ill. The only remaining critters were Mrs. Nickels the cat and a dog named Gladys.

There would be no more morning meetings over coffee and homemade rolls. All the farm hands were retired or had moved onto working farms. Now the only thing left were empty chairs and memories. Sadness was the only guest that lingered.

Hugh was tired. It showed on his face and in the slow way he moved his tall, frail body about the kitchen to prepare tea. It was clear that what little energy he had was reserved for the woman he loved with all his heart, the woman he vowed to care for so many years ago in a small country church on the vast open prairie. The same church his parents had married in.

That church still stands, but it's no longer a church—nor is there a prairie surrounding it. There are no more country weddings, baptisms, or funerals. No longer can you hear the singing that once seeped out of its cracks.

Now it's an office building for the housing development that swallowed up the land. Hundreds of look-alike houses with no personality have now consumed what was once rolling prairies and bountiful farmland.

So many farmers were drunk on the idea of how much money they were being offered by the developers. Honestly, no one blamed them for it. For them, it meant no more back breaking work, no more depending on the weather for everything. Farming is physically taxing, and every new season is a gamble. A seasoned farmer had to read the weather by the smell of the earth, because his life and that of his family were contingent on it.

No, no one blamed them for selling. There were, however, a few who didn't. They simply could not imagine the lump sum cash was worth leaving the lands that had been in their families for generations. Money could not replace being able to stand on their porch every morning and evening to take in the smell of the earth. Predawn void of a rooster's call to remind them to get the coffee brewing. Living so close to another's home that you couldn't pee outside or run around naked if you chose was just inconceivable. Most of all, they couldn't imagine anyone telling them what to do with their land—ever. Few families in the county had resisted the offers from developers. Hugh and Betty were among those few.

It's true that farming is a hard way to make a living, but it's an honest living—rewarding those who do it with freedom every single day. This was Hugh and Betty Roberts' world, and they simply couldn't imagine any other way of life. So, they stayed put.

Hugh and Betty had always believed their son, Charly, would take over the family farm, build a house, and raise a family of his own on the land. But soon after graduating from high school, he went off to college to become a veterinarian. Although during his seven years of schooling he was home each summer for a couple of months to help out, his studies and resulting career had taken priority.

It wasn't a complete surprise to Hugh and Betty that he wanted to become a veterinarian. Ever since he was able to walk, he played doctor with the animals around the farm. Charly was not afraid to swipe his mother's meat thermometer from the kitchen drawer to maneuver it up a pig's butt to take its temperature. He'd even tackle calves to the ground when he was no taller than they were so he could wrap a towel around their heads, claiming they had mumps and needed treatment. His imaginary skills went on through childhood and would eventually evolve into a teaching job at Iowa State University, 115 miles north of the Roberts farm in their hometown of Ottumwa.

Hugh and Betty were proud that Charly was doing what he'd always dreamed of, even though they knew that one day the farm would become too much work for just the two of them. Selling was out of the question, so they decided to lease out their fields to other farmers. Thousands of acres of corn and beans would now be the responsibility of someone else and collecting annual checks while retaining their land would be easier than working the soil themselves.

Life took on an easy pace. In the mornings, before the sun climbed the riverbanks, Hugh and Evert—his friend of over fifty years—fished the arms of the river running through the rolling farmland. They caught whatever they could, only to release them back into the murky waters.

Betty divided her time between volunteering at their church and spending time with the farm animals. She preferred being outside, happily feeding and tending to the livestock. It wasn't uncommon to walk into the barn and hear a one-sided conversation between Betty and a cow or some other four-legged creature. But once she started naming the hogs and the beef cows, the butchering came to an abrupt halt—as did any future sales. Even the eggs collected daily didn't go up for sale. Instead, she gave them away to the local food shelf or to others who wanted or needed them.

Eventually Hugh accepted that the critters who lived there were a part of the family and no longer a means of making a living. Whatever made Betty happy, made Hugh happy. But that happy time was short-lived.

THE DEMON DEMENTIA

Hugh sat the steaming cups of tea down on the table and lowered his six-foot frame to sit alongside his wife. He watched her stare into the worn, old wallpaper, lost and in another world, a place beyond the walls his great grandfather built.

She didn't speak or acknowledge his presence. She rarely did anymore. It was something he didn't think he would ever get used to, and the brief joy of hearing her utter the word *Boy* just minutes before had already left his heart.

The afternoon sun shone through the front window, warming the room to a cozy temperature, but also magnifying the food stains on her dress. He could smell the urine that seeped through her full diaper, and he was ashamed of himself.

All her life, his wife had taken pride in the way she kept herself and her home. He used to call her his "shiny penny," but those days were long gone. Now he was tired of the wrestling matches and the terror on her face as he changed her clothes or bathed her little body. Too often it was easier for him to leave her dirty.

Hugh received frequent offers of assistance from the women at their church—the newer Lutheran church in town. The one that they were no longer able to attend. Once or twice a week he'd get a call from one of the ladies offering to clean the home, bathe his wife, or simply sit with her for a few hours to give him a break he desperately needed but always refused—not always out of pride, but fear.

He knew that everyone was a stranger to her—even himself—and he didn't want to risk scaring her any more than she already was. Even so, looking at her grimy state made him heartsick, like so many other things that broke his heart over the past ten years.

So be it, Hugh thought. They would drink their tea, and then he would muster up the courage to give her a bath. In his heart he knew that she loved him, no matter what, and in this moment that's all that mattered to him.

He hoped to stimulate a past reflex by lifting the rim of the teacup to her lips. He was satisfied when she turned away from the wallpaper and used her bony hand to hold the cup by herself. He kept his large hand nearby as she took an apprehensive drink of the lukewarm liquid then quickly pulled it away. A look of pain flashed across her face, like she'd just burned her lips, but he knew full well that the tea was far from hot. He played along, apologizing and taking the cup out of her hand. When he sat the tea on the table, she bent her head way down near the cup and then turned her face upwards, directly under him. The action was innocent and childlike, and it made him smile.

"You silly willy," he said to her, playfully. "Would you like some more tea?"

"No," she answered clearly, straightening herself up in the chair. "I want Boy."

Other than that morning outside, she hadn't spoken a word in many months. Now she'd used several in a sentence and he could only stare at her, shocked. Any second she would return to the wallpaper world, so he didn't dare look away.

Wife stood and pointed towards the window. "I want Boy," she repeated.

He quickly stood and grabbed her waist to steady her. She pulled at his shirt sleeve, pleading silently for him to walk her to the window. He knew this moment wouldn't last but was grateful for it just the same.

He shuffled her across the creaky green linoleum floor, and by the time they reached the ray of sun coming through the window, it had happened. She was gone again—blank—back into the world he couldn't enter.

It was over, and he was angry at himself for being disappointed. Ashamed to have expected more, hoped for more. He'd promised God a long time ago that he would accept what came his way and be appreciative for what he still had. And he *was* grateful, but he was tired and empty as well.

Hugh sat Betty down in the nearest chair, a worn leather recliner that was easy to get her in and out of. "Would you like some more tea?"

There was no response, no recognition. He really hadn't expected any but talking to her was a routine— one he would never quit.

He stood at the edge of the chair and watched as the stream of sunlight worked its magic on Betty's face. She quickly closed her eyes and fell asleep. She was safe now. *Lucky booger,* he thought with a tinge of guilt. Then, in the quiet of his home, he announced to no one that he was going to go run her a bath.

Hugh sat on the floor and watched the water fill their old bathtub, letting his mind wander back to all the times he had bathed his little boy in this very tub. The giggling, the splashing, and the occasional crying from soapy eyes played out in his mind's eye.

He remembered how he would wrap his little boy up in a towel and carry him in to see his mama so she could give him the smell test, cracking them up as she sniffed his neck, arms, and feet, tickling him as she went along.

Those were happy times, and even though he did his best to stay out of the past, he couldn't help himself. He hungered for those years and accepted that where the good memories rested, so did the sad ones. The ones he had to remember for the both of them. The ones that now ate him alive.

ONE BOY LOST

It was nine years ago that Hugh bathed his son for the last time. Charly was thirty-one years old and weighed only eighty-nine pounds—his hollow blue eyes never leaving his father's as he was washed.

Hugh wrapped his son in a towel, like he did when he was a boy, and carried the man he'd raised to the couch, tucking in blankets gently around him.

Betty sat on one end of the couch, stroking Charley's face and hair into the night while Hugh took the other end, feverishly beseeching God.

Cancer won. Charly took his last breath at 1:35 am. Numb and silent, neither Hugh nor Betty left the couch until morning came through the window. Only then did they reluctantly let go of the most important person in their world.

The grief that followed was blinding. Hugh was drowning in it, and therefore, didn't notice what was happening to his Betty. Little by little, the invisible monster called dementia was swallowing her up.

Hugh hung his large body over the bath water and cried like a baby at the memories. Trying his best to muffle the sobs that escaped his mouth, he grabbed a towel and buried his face until he felt something warm rub against him. He looked down to see their cat, Mrs. Nickels, staring up at him. She'd found her way in through the open door and her greenish-black eyes were asking, "Hold me?" He sat back on his feet. She crawled into his large lap and began to purr. Hugh dropped the towel and picked up Mrs. Nickels, who instantly nestled into his neck. Soaking up the sound of her heartbeat, he whispered, "Thank you."

Mrs. Nickels and the chickens were now all they had left of the animals. It was the creatures on the farm that had finally set off the alarm bells in Hugh's head, warning him that something was wrong with his wife. Betty had always taken great pride in her pets, making sure they had full bellies and clean coats. But Hugh had to accept she was no longer capable when hungry cats would lace between his legs and pigs would stray from open pens. The day he found her wandering aimlessly down the dirt road outside the house—confused and distraught—he took over the feeding and watering, taking her with him each time.

But even that had become too difficult to keep up. He couldn't take his eyes off her or she would vanish into thin air. Sometimes he'd find her around a corner, talking to herself or staring off into nothingness. Other times he'd rush around the farm calling her name in a panic. Several times she'd gone missing for so long he'd had to enlist the help of others to find her.

Eventually, Hugh decided to give the rest of the animals away, refusing any money offered to him. He gave the hogs to Evert Heins—his friend and neighbor to the east, and a good old boy he'd known since grade school.

The beef cattle he sent over to his western neighbors—Fara Kremer and her brothers, Chod and Dude. They'd been friends since the beginning of time, it seemed. Afterwards, both neighbors made sure to show their appreciation by giving the Roberts more than enough butchered meat to sustain an army. Finally, Gladys, the Roberts little cocker spaniel, just disappeared one day.

ANOTHER BOY FOUND

With Mrs. Nickels hanging over his shoulder, Hugh turned off the water and walked into the living room, fully prepared to coax his wife to her waiting bath. It took him a minute to realize that the chair and room were empty. Mrs. Nickels scratched his arm while jumping from his grasp. She took off through the living room like she was on fire, running past the empty chair, into the kitchen and out the open door. Frantic, Hugh called his wife's name as he followed the cat outside.

He dashed to the closest building: the chicken coop. Nothing there but chickens. Then he ran to the barn—empty and echoing her name as he called it. He rushed to the stables and then to the stock yard. Nothing.

Where could she be? he thought as he stood in his driveway, searching the length of the gravel road and seeing only a cloud of dust that the wind swept across. "Betty!" he called, startling a red fox digging in the ditch nearby. He called over and over as he ran through the yard and around to the front of the house. Tripping on the fallen flower boxes, he grabbed at the corner of the siding to keep from going down.

Breathless, he leaned on the corner of the house and that's when he saw her, sitting under the large oak tree next to the bird they'd found that morning. As relief washed over him it was replaced by anxiety. He felt worn thin and questioned just how long he could physically keep this up.

There was no hurry now that he could see her. She was safe, so he continued to lean against the house, catching his breath and letting his old heart slow down a bit.

Betty sat cross-legged on a blanket of leaves; stringy gray hair splayed over her cheek as she tipped her head forward. Hugh was amazed at her flexibility, considering her age. He watched her lean over the dead bird as her mouth began to move, like she was talking to it. But then he realized the truth of what he saw.

She *was* talking to it!

He pushed himself away from the house and cautiously approached her from the side. When he was close enough, he discovered she wasn't talking to the damn bird—she was singing to it!

Hugh watched as she rocked her body from side to side in sync with the lullaby coming from her sweet mouth. He looked down to the dead bird to find it looking back at him—clearly very much alive.

He was surprised the little thing had survived, recalling the loud thud it made when hitting the window. Plus, he knew how birds were one of Mrs. Nickel's favorite meals, and he wondered over how the cat hadn't gobbled it up by now.

Betty stopped singing and looked up at her husband. Another strong breeze swept across the field and into the yard, rummaging through her hair and lifting the floral fabric over her lap. Combined with the intense look on her face, the wind made her look a bit like a mad scientist in a polyester dress.

The singing stopped and Betty pointed at the bird, saying clearly, "Boy." Hugh didn't know what the fascination with the bird was and frankly didn't care. His wife was trying to communicate with him, which was all he was concerned about.

Hugh looked around at the dark clouds, sensing an oncoming storm. He decided it might be a good idea if he brought them both into the house.

BOY

I thought I was having a bad dream or a kind of déjà vu when I woke to the sound of leaves being crushed. Before I could look around, there she was again—the same shell of a woman from before. This time she sat down next to me, singing, and gagging me with her scent. I wondered why she was there. More than that, I wondered how the sound of something so beautiful and so calming could come from something so terribly stinky.

Then the sweet sound stopped, and I was being lifted by a huge hand—scooped into the sky so quickly I thought my heart and stomach would drop out over the side. The hand was attached to the tall, strong one: The Old Man. With my body completely covered I couldn't see what was happening. I ached and pooped myself, fearing what would happen next. But the deep voice I heard was tender as he explained to the empty shell of a woman that rain was on its way, and that they needed to take me into the house where it was warm. A little voice repeated, "Warm."

THE RESCUER AND THE RESCUED

A curious Mrs. Nickels appeared at their feet as Hugh and Betty wound their way through the fallen leaves to the house. The parade came through the kitchen and continued into the open dining and living room area where Betty automatically sat down at the table. Still holding the bird in one hand, Hugh walked the few feet back to the kitchen to grab a dish towel. When he turned back towards the table, he saw his wife and Mrs. Nickels each scrutinizing him curiously from their own dining chairs. Hugh grinned and thought maybe it was time they all had lunch.

By the time he retraced the few feet to the table, Betty's left hand was stroking the attentive cat. *What had awoken within her?* Hugh didn't know and didn't care exactly what was happening because at this moment his table had a lunch guest, and he was going to enjoy every second of it.

With his free hand, Hugh quickly made a nest out of a towel that wife had embroidered years ago. The sewed-on image of a cow and the name 'Daisy' were faded but still visible. He laid the bird down in the middle of the towel. Knowing full well that one of his guests would be very happy to have the little guy for lunch, he bent over and picked up the shoe box that doubled as a file drawer. Turning it upside down, he emptied years' worth of bank statements onto the floor.

Before he could sit down and transfer the bird, Betty had already cupped the towel in her hands and carefully set it into the box. Hugh stood looking at her in disbelief. He hadn't expected her to remain in his world for so long. Fact is, he didn't expect anything anymore. He wished he had timed her attention span, her here and now, whatever that was. But right now he didn't need his trusty Timex to know that this was the longest period in many months that a part of her remained lucid. She was there with him, and he was enjoying every precious second.

The loud grumble of his stomach snapped him out of his thoughts, out of his state of disbelief. Hoping Betty could remain long enough for him warm the soup and make tuna sandwiches, he left for the kitchen, keeping a watchful eye on her and the attentive Mrs. Nickels.

The worst that could happen was that Betty would fade back into the wallpaper, and Mrs. Nickels would eat their guest.

As he prepared their plates, he remembered the waiting bath. It could continue to wait. Everything else could wait.

Without incident, Betty accepted the spoonfuls of warm bean soup and the bite-size sandwich held up to her mouth by Hugh. *So far so good*, he thought. Mrs. Nickels sat upright in the adjacent chair, following the action by moving her head back and forth from the box to the large handfuls of goodness that moved across the table. She never made a move for either, causing Hugh to wonder if the cat could sense the small miracle unfolding before them. He also questioned whether he was losing his mind by imagining what the cat was thinking.

In between feeding Betty her bites of lunch, Hugh took bites of his own, seriously considering his state of mind. It wasn't that long ago that he had pleaded with God to end their lives, to end the hell on earth they were in. He'd woke the next day, disappointed by their still beating hearts. That's when the thought had crept in. It wouldn't even be that hard to do. He had enough pills for the both of them. And he could turn on the gas and leave it on. Yes, he knew ways.

The only thing that kept him from acting on his desperation was the hope of seeing their son again, in heaven. He believed that if he ended their lives by his own hand, heaven's doors would be closed to him.

Watching his wife now, he shuddered at the memory, and guilt rode heavy on his aging shoulders.

BOY

Okay, so there I was lying in a damn shoe box, carried away from my view of the sky, carried away from the squirrels and the safety of the large tree. I shouldn't have lollygagged in the sunshine. I should have ignored my pain and tried to fly away when I had the chance, but it's too late now.

Now I am a prisoner, and I am afraid. I look into the faces that surround me, especially the furry one with hungry eyes, and swear that if I ever get back to into the open air I will escape.

BOX

From a hiding spot, Hugh took out a pair of scissors and began making holes in the lid of the box. He was fairly certain the air holes would be fruitless, but he didn't think his wife could handle watching Mrs. Nickels eat her "Boy" alive. Honestly, he didn't think he could watch that either. They'd had enough death. Nope, when the bird died, as he was certain it would, it would do so under the lid of the shoe box. Then he would toss it outside for his Mrs. Nickels to carry away.

Anticipating the tide to change, Hugh seized the moment by cleaning up the dirty dishes. He admired the beautiful old wood as he polished the vacant area of the table, thinking someday soon he'd tackle the piles of paper that cluttered most its surface. He winced at the dumping ground it had become.

When he was done cleaning up, Hugh put the lid on the box and said, "Time for this little fellow to get some sleep." Looking at his wife he added, "And time for you to take a bath." He held his breath and waited for resistance, but none came. She merely pushed her chair from the table, and with wobbly legs, stood up waiting for his trusted hands to guide her.

Mrs. Nickels was no longer interested and jumped down from her chair for another seat on the couch.

On the way to the bathroom, Betty suddenly put on the brakes. *Here it comes,* Hugh thought, anticipating the familiar and painful wrestling match. But there wasn't one. She simply turned her head back towards the table and pointed. Not waiting for more—afraid of breaking the spell—he maneuvered her around and backtracked to the table, picking up the box before taking her to the waiting bath. He set the box down on the closed toilet seat while he undressed his wife.

Rivulets dribbled from the soapy cloth, and water beads made a noisy, liquid echo as they plopped into the surface of the bath. Even though it was the only sound, the near silence didn't haunt Hugh with sadness the way it had earlier. He no longer felt quite as alone in the same room with his wife because her eyes were alive and sparkling with contentment. She was so captivated by the little box on the toilet seat lid that she didn't seem to notice as he moved the cloth over her withered body. Sometimes she would even crane her neck to look around her husband when his large frame interrupted her gaze.

Hugh felt his own version of contentment; all was good in the Roberts home for now. The only thing he wished for right then was that he had time to spare and to share it with someone.

By the time the bath was over, they both smelled of soap—a scent almost as good as Hugh felt. He dressed her in a fresh cotton dress as he wondered where her mind was. Although she didn't wear the blank stare he was accustom to, she wouldn't look at him either. Her attention was still on the box, which now sat on their dresser.

Was there magic in that box? "Silly man," he said out loud. Hugh didn't want to press his luck, but at the same time thought that maybe, just maybe, it would be a good time to feed the chickens. He'd forgotten them in all the morning excitement.

He wanted to take Betty with him. Lord knew they could both use some fresh air. If the rain held off, they could walk the long driveway to the mailbox, turn around, and call it a day—a good one at that.

These had become chores he did in a rush while Betty napped after breakfast. He no longer enjoyed them because he practically had to run as he did them, always eager to return to the house before she woke up, fearful of what could happen during those fifteen minutes he would be gone.

The driveway was a quarter mile long, and because of his fear and anxiety, he no longer walked it but drove his pickup or four-wheeler instead.

"How about we go outside?" he asked his quiet companion, helping her up from the side of the bed. He added a soft, worn sweater to her shoulders, just in case.

Quick on the draw, her arm shot up and pointed towards the dresser.

"Of course, we can't forget the bird," he said.

"Boy!" she quickly corrected him.

Smiling, he grabbed the box from the dresser and handed it to her.

"Okay, Boy," he said, and out into the late afternoon they went.

Betty held onto the box tightly as her husband went to work. She was the keeper of it for now, standing in the small space of the chicken coop and watching his every move through the doorway with an expression on her face that he couldn't place. It wasn't one he'd seen before or at least not one he'd seen in an awfully long time.

In a messy haphazard pattern, he threw the meal down outside the coop and Betty made no effort to walk away so he stole a few extra minutes to shovel out the old straw and replace it with new.

On both sides of the driveway there were fields of corn, now harvested. Even in the wind you could hear the pheasants running through the few dry stalks that remained. The distant fence lines stood like loyal soldiers waiting for the day they could come home. The air smelled wet and of dirt, the scent one becomes addicted to after having lived off the land.

As they walked the long driveway arm in arm, Hugh got a whiff of his childhood. All around him he smelled the seventy-eight years of his life. He turned to look at his wife who still clung protectively to the small box and wondered whether she too could smell memories in the wind.

The rain looked like it was still miles away, but the wind was strong and present. In Iowa, the wind is never far away—always sneaking around, reminding you of how pointless it was to comb your hair or wear a cap.

By the time they reached the mailbox it had started to sprinkle. Hugh let go of Betty's arm long enough to retrieve the mail and shove it inside his flannel shirt, when a gust of wind swept by them, taking with it the lid from the box. Across one field and into the next it tumbled, until being captured by the loyal soldiers.

A shriek escaped Betty's mouth; her reaction unexpectedly quick. Before Hugh knew what was happening, she grabbed the bird from the box and stuck it in her dress, tucking it between her breast and bra, which smelled of soap. Then, with a devious grin, she lifted the box up and let go. Out into the fields it went.

BOY

I bounced around in the dark—dizzy and sick—for what seemed like forever. I rolled and crashed, the cloth nest twisting around my face and suffocating me until the jostling suddenly stopped. Dark skies appeared overhead, and a rush of air blew in all around me. I could taste freedom, but I wasn't ready! I hadn't expected the chance of escape so soon.

Rain pelted my face, making it impossible for me to see, and before I could think of a plan, Wife's hand encircled me. I could hear the protest from Old Man as she put me inside her dress, next to her body in some other nest. It was warm and I could breathe, but I feared I was trapped much worse than before.

CONNECTION

They were almost to the house when Betty veered sharply to the right, pulling Hugh back towards the chicken coop. Rain was now more than a sprinkle, running down their faces and matting their hair to their foreheads. As the rain ran down his weathered face and neck, Hugh remembered another time before Charly, before marriage, before the years had carved their lives and before sadness knew who they were.

THEN

That morning after racing through his chores, a young Hugh Roberts biked the eight miles to Betty's house to help her finish all hers. The long ride down the gravel roads in the blistering heat was always worth it. Other than at school or church, it was the only time he could see her—the only time he was allowed to be alone with her. Rules for young adults were so different then.

They were in the chicken coop collecting eggs when the rain came. Betty held the basket tightly to her waist, and when the first thunder roared, she jumped, dropping the basket to the ground, breaking all the gathered eggs.

With good intentions, the two of them got down on their hands and knees to pick up the shells and slime that covered everything, including some of the chickens. They laughed at the impossible feat of completing the chore as Betty's long brown hair brushed against Hugh's shoulders. That's when he leaned forward and pressed his mouth against her perfect pink lips for the first time.

Hugh was startled when she stood up and ran out into the rain, thinking she was running away from him. But his dismay disappeared when he saw her dance and twirl under the falling drops, pulling him out with her until they were both soaked to the bone. She was no longer afraid of the thunder and lightning or the scolding that was sure to come from her mother. That's when he knew that she was the one for him.

NOW

Betty pulled on Hugh's arm, beckoning him to follow her lead, bringing him back to the here and now—wherever that was. She pulled him into the chicken coop, where the rain made music on the tin roof.

He could tell by the vacant look on her face that she didn't know what to do once inside, so he sat two wooden crates on end, making a seat for them both.

They sat facing the rows of nesting chickens, listening to the cooing and the pounding rain. What was left of the afternoon light came through the two little windows on each side of the building. Soon it would be dark outside, but Hugh didn't care. He was in no hurry.

He peeked at her from the corner of his eye, wishing he could steal one more kiss from those lips, but he didn't dare. He didn't want to frighten her. Even though she was the one who led them there, he couldn't count on it being because of anything she remembered.

Once total darkness and regret for what was no more had washed over Hugh, he guided her back into the house to dry off and have some supper.

Hugh didn't dare ask about the bird in her bra. He couldn't be sure she still knew it was there. He assumed that it was smothered by now. The thought of it wedged against the skin of her breast disgusted him, but at the same time he knew that—dead or alive—taking it from her was going to be tricky.

The past year, Betty's memory had dissolved to complete dust, as did her ability to feed and dress herself or take care of any of her bathroom needs—or anything else for that matter. Her memory prior was poor at best, but she would have moments of clarity, which kept Hugh going. That and his love for her.

When they first learned that she had dementia, a friend had given them a movie, suggesting that it would be an opportune time for them to see it.

The movie was a beautiful but sad, romantic portrayal of dementia. It was about a husband who altered his life for his sick wife, and for her wonderful moments of clarity. It was about the commitment two people make to each other and the journey that commitment took them on.

Hugh took that commitment very seriously, however, because of the sugar coating in that particular movie and a little denial, he banked on the possibility of such clarity with his wife. He walked away from the movie with an unrealistic view of what was to come, which created even more anxiety and disappointment. Wife walked away from it angry and more afraid than she had ever been in her entire life.

Once she was officially diagnosed, it all seemed to happen so fast, or at least that's what he told himself. He chose not to recognize that for years he'd been covering up what she wasn't capable of doing or knowing or remembering. By the time he acknowledged it was a disease and not just grief or normal forgetfulness, she was in the thick of it, depending on him for almost everything.

The worst parts were the unexpected bursts of anger and the combative way she fought him. He could live with all else but having to restrain his wife is what broke his heart.

After finishing up the rest of the bean soup and the peanut butter crackers he'd added to their dinner menu, he cleared the table and returned from the kitchen with a wet cloth to clean Betty's face and hands. She looked up and held out her hand when he approached, which Hugh automatically put into his own.

Betty shook her head from side to side, freeing her hand from his, and holding it out again. Curious, he gave her the towel and watched as she wiped off the table. When she was done, she handed it back to him and went into the bedroom by herself.

Smiling at the towel, he said, "Okay then, let's get ready for bed!"

He hurried after her, still nervous about meeting resistance over the nighttime routine. However, there was no incident as he changed her into her nighties, removing the still, little bird from her bra, then covering her up in her own little nest of quilts. He could feel her eyes on his back as he carried the bird to the dresser. He could also feel the tiny heart beating against his hand.

"Tough little booger," he mumbled as he opened the top drawer. "I'll put him on my handkerchief so he'll be as comfy as you are. In the morning we'll all have breakfast together. How's that sound?"

When no argument came, he laid the bird on his stack of folded hankies, turning it over so it was on its back.

The bird's eyes opened, and although he knew it was absurd to think that the creature was studying him—even listening to him—that's how it seemed. Did the bird understand the word *breakfast*? Did it know that he might not see the morning light?

Hugh closed the drawer, feeling kind of sorry for the damn thing. When he turned around, he was surprised to see Mrs. Nickels nestled in alongside Betty, who still wore smudges of peanut butter on her face. Her left hand had found its way out from underneath the quilt to stroke the sneaky cat. Hugh knew the cat was no dummy; she smelled the peanut butter. It was an easy treat he was certain she would have as soon as he left the room.

Before turning off the lights, Hugh glanced at the drawer to be sure he'd closed it. Satisfied the cat wouldn't be having the bird as well as peanut butter, he said, "Good night, you guys."

Once he was alone the living room, he said aloud, "Lord, whatever it is that you gave us today, I sure would appreciate you bringing it back tomorrow."

Then he sat down and fell fast asleep in his chair, dreaming of his boy, Charly. He dreamt of that awful day Charly came down the driveway, alone and unexpected, in the brown truck that read "Iowa State University" on its doors.

BOY

I could tell by the way he looked into my eyes that he was onto me. Old Man knew I was planning an escape! When the light came back, I would have to act, but first I planned to dream of what he called "breakfast."

THEN

Hugh had made plans to meet Evert and his son Mike at the river later that day. They were going to search for arrowheads along the bank, something they did often after the spring rains. Arrowheads were one of the few things Hugh collected, and he had accrued quite the assortment.

Betty was in the back of the house putting away the clean laundry she'd just pulled off the clothesline and Hugh was at the kitchen sink, cleaning up after breakfast when Charly came driving up.

Hugh's eyebrows knit together as he watched the morning sun bouncing off the silver bumper. He was sure it wasn't Charly's day off—he knew his son's schedule well. He worried that maybe Charly had been laid off or—even worse—fired from his job. But that was unlikely. His son was a hard worker, and everyone loved him at the school. Hugh continued to speculate, because whatever the reason his son had come unannounced was something worth driving an hour and a half for. When Charly put the truck in park, Hugh figured he'd know the answer soon enough, but instead, he got out of his truck and headed straight to the barn.

Boy

Maybe he needs to borrow something, Hugh thought, forcing his attention away from the window and finishing up the dishes. The kitchen was spotless, and quite a bit of time had passed with still no sign of Charly when Hugh finally gave into his curiosity. He walked outside and into the barn where the daylight and dust mixed together, blinding him until his eyes could adjust to the light. The sound of sobbing stopped him cold.

Focusing through the dust, he saw his grown son sitting in a stall on a pile of straw next to Bob, the bull Charly had raised from a baby. The bull had been born with defected rear legs, making them much shorter than the front ones, and rendering it worthless on the market. Hugh had planned on putting the animal down shortly after discovering the defect, but Charly and his mother pleaded with him to spare the goofy looking critter, promising that they would care for him, which they happily did.

Hugh stood frozen against an old post, listening to his boy—a full grown man—cry and talk to Bob. Charly had always been an attractive kid—blond hair, blue eyes, and medium build. But now his body looked so small lying over his 450-pound friend.

"I'm sorry," Charly blubbered to the bull. "I'm so sorry."

Hugh couldn't take it any longer. He pushed his lean body away from the post and knelt quietly down on the straw next to Bob, across from his son.

"Hey buddy," Hugh said, keeping his voice soft. "What's goin' on here?"

With swollen eyes, Charly sat up and looked across the bull to his father, snot and tears mixing as they ran onto Bob. The animal had one large brown eye focused intently on Charly, his strong tail flipping up and down, stirring a cloud of dust around them.

"I'm dying, Dad," Charly blurted. "I'm dying."

Hugh placed his hands on Bob's belly to steady himself. "What do you mean, son? I don't understand . . . how could you be . . . dying?"

Charly wiped his nose on his sleeve, sighed, and said, "I've been having some trouble with my balance the past few months," his voice faltered, and he searched for his father's eyes. "My left leg doesn't want to move on its own, I have to drag it behind me."

A moan escaped Hugh's mouth. Charly reached across Bob's huge rib cage for his father's large hands and said, "I was sure it was nothing, that's why I didn't call you and mom. But then my headaches started, so Eileen talked me into going to one of our colleagues at work, just to ask some questions . . . so I did."

Eileen was Charly's part time girlfriend—part time only because they were both committed to their jobs at the university, not because they weren't committed to each other. Their shift work made a personal life nearly impossible, but somehow, they managed because the second part of the news Charly had brought home with him that day was that Eileen was pregnant.

Hugh held tightly to his son's hands, afraid to let go, afraid to hear more. The horrible silence of the barn was broken only when Bob farted. Hugh and his son couldn't help but crack up.

They sat on the damp ground looking across at one another when their laughing morphed into a chorus of crying.

From outside they heard, "Hugh, where in the hell are you?"

They stood up and walked away from Bob, hand in hand, ignoring the sound his strong tail made as it slapped the ground in protest. They went through the open barn doors and away from the place Charly had chosen to run, away from the safety and sanity he had known would be in there for him.

When Betty came into view, they stopped walking. She knew right away something was terribly wrong; she could tell by the way her men held onto each other and the raw agony on her baby's face. She fell to the ground at their feet and began praying to God.

Charly bent over and touched his mother's shoulder, interrupting her prayers by saying softly,

"Mom, I have something I want to talk to you about." Before she could respond he added, "Don't you worry about God, I've already talked to him. Now it's time I talk to you and Dad. How about we go to the house so you can make us some coffee and warm up some of those sweet rolls I know you've got hiding in there?"

That brought a half smile to her ashen face. If you are a woman from generations past, you know that food represents more than just a meal. It represents love and togetherness, the energy spent cooking, baking, and brewing coming straight from the heart. Your world and those in it revolve around the constant presence and preparation of a home-cooked meal. It is a lesson these women learned without being told by their mothers and grandmothers. Feeding their people gave them purpose, and more times than not that very food could cure most any woe . . . almost any.

Distracted by his request, Betty stood up and wiped the dust from her dress. She looked from Hugh to Charly, searching for an explanation. When none came, she replied, "Of course, honey. Let's get you to the house so mama can put some meat on your bones."

Huge winced at the words she'd spoken as they followed her into the house—into the cozy kitchen that smelled of home. Into the place that would never be the same.

Betty warmed the rolls and brewed a fresh pot of coffee, avoiding the eyes at the table. She chatted mindlessly about the new calf born a few days before and how it hadn't wanted to suckle from its mother. "Today it's sucking like a pro, thank goodness." She went on and on about the calf until the coffee pot went silent. Then she went silent. As if in a trance, she watched the steam rise from the cups as she filled them at the counter. For the first time in her life she was afraid to move, afraid to look at her two men sitting at the table.

"Mom," Charly said, bringing her back to the task at hand.

"Just a second," she said, but before picking up the cups she reached over and grabbed the cross that for years hung above their kitchen sink and slid it into her dress pocket.

Once Betty sat down, Hugh reached for her hand under the table and squeezed it, conveying that everything was going to be all right and to give Charly the floor.

She forced herself to be calm and quiet and ended up staring at his curly blond hair—way too long for a man his age she thought. His eyes were like his father's—so blue you could paint the sky with the color. Her son was simply beautiful.

Charly began talking, tying his hair behind his head which made her chuckle inappropriately.

"I'm going to tell you guys the good news first okay?" Hugh looked down at his lap where his wife's hand had returned the squeeze. Looking across at her, he knew in his heart that whatever was to be they would survive it as a team.

"Eileen and I planned on telling you this together, but she couldn't be here today, so here it goes." Taking a sip of coffee, Charly continued, "We're getting married as soon as possible, and we would really like it if we could get married here on the farm."

A squeal shot out of Betty's mouth, but before she could say anything, Charly held out his hand as if to say wait, there's more—and there was. "I know you won't approve of the order of this, but Eileen is pregnant, three months pregnant."

Betty put both hands over her mouth, as if to prevent both the joy and judgment from spilling out.

"We didn't plan on it happening like this. We'd talked about getting married in the fall and then later start a family. We talked about Eileen taking a sabbatical once she became pregnant since we make pretty good money and can easily live on one income. That was the plan anyway. Obviously now things have changed. I'm sorry mom, it wasn't supposed to happen this way."

Betty got up and ran around to her grown baby, nearly smothering him in her arms. "I don't care about the order, honey. What I care about is you and Eileen and having grand babies!" She released her hands from around his neck and raised them to the air in a "praise the Lord" gesture. "Hugh, did you hear that? We're going to be grandparents!" With the widest of grins, she bent over and kissed Hugh square on the lips. "Praise the Lord and thank you, Jesus!"

"Mom, would you mind getting me a hot bun and some butter? I think I need some fuel for the next part," Charly said, giving his father a quick glance.

"Of course, honey," Betty said, spinning on her heels.

Now, it was Hugh's turn to look into his son's blue eyes. They looked back at him with fear and sadness. He said nothing as he reached over and squeezed his son's arm in support.

Charly stuffed his mouth with the homemade goodness, taking periodic sips of coffee, then shoving more sweet bread in—prolonging the moment of truth. When he could eat no more, he faced his audience, who waited like Paul Harvey's listeners for "the rest of the story."

Clearing his throat, Charly said, "We—me, Eileen, and the baby—would like to move here . . . home . . . if we could. And as soon as possible."

Betty no longer had a sense of any bad news, the notion forgotten and replaced by the good news which she didn't think could get any better. When she started to get out of her chair to jump for joy or thank Jesus one more time, Hugh took hold of her arm—a silent warning.

Confused by Hugh's reprimand, Betty blurted, "Of course you two—I mean you three—can move home! Nothing would make this old gal happier. When can you—?"

Charly cut her off with, "Mom there's still more. I've been having health issues the past few months."

Betty shook her head in denial and tried to interrupt.

"Please mom, this isn't easy."

Betty felt like she might throw up, but she kept quiet, listening raptly to her son's symptoms. If she were honest with herself, she'd known there was something wrong with Charly well before today. She could see it in the way he walked, the exhaustion in his face.

"I told the doctor my symptoms and she immediately ordered a CAT scan, an MRI, and a series of blood tests, which I completed last week," Charly explained. "I was too afraid to meet at her office to go over the results, so I asked that she fax them to me instead. I got them this morning. I have a brain tumor and I'll be lucky to live long enough to see my child born." He took another deep breath. "I haven't even told Eileen; I just jumped in my truck and came home."

Hugh watched the color drain from his wife's face as Charly pulled the papers out from the inside of his jacket and laid them on the table.

"You can read them if you want, but the doctor says it's inoperable, the prognosis is grim." His face crumbled before he fell against the table and wept.

The second Charly put a period at the end of his last sentence, Betty threw up all over the table, the top of Charly's head and the papers she had no intention of ever reading.

A month later, Charly and Eileen had quit their jobs, emptied out their houses, and moved what items they wanted to keep to the farm.

On July 8, 2006, with a few friends and Eileen's family at their side, they married in the old red barn on the Roberts farm. Pastor Dale from the Good Shepard Lutheran Church presided over them. If he judged the obvious lump Eileen carried in the front of the simple white dress she wore, he didn't let it be known.

It was a small, beautiful wedding—all about the couple. Everyone that loved and cared for them made sure of that. Eliza Reeve, a friend of the Roberts from church, had spent the entire morning in the Iowa heat picking wheelbarrows full of prairie flowers and grasses. The shade of the barn was refreshingly cool as she and a giddy Betty decorated the stall doors and makeshift pulpit. Along the floor and next to the folding chairs, they sat wooden barrels that overflowed with sweet grass and early wheat, blending appropriately with the lingering smell of manure and hay. Blue ribbons hung from the rafters and the hay loft, doves perched in between the decorations, cooing as if they were hired to do so. It was perfect.

Bob was present, at Charly's request, along with Gladys and Daisy and—scampering around at everyone's feet—a pregnant Mary Bell, Mrs. Nickel's mother. There wasn't enough room in the barn for all the critters their son invited, so Hugh moved most of them out to the stockyard until the party was over.

The air was still thick with humidity as the sun went down for the day. Captured in its moisture was the aroma of growing fields, remnants of a roasted pig, and the lingering embers from the bonfire that had blazed throughout the celebration.

Once the guests had gone, and the bride and groom had disappeared for the night, Hugh and Betty were alone again.

Hugh retired to the house with a weary shuffle, pooped out after the festivities and the chore of having to return the critters to the barn. Betty had stayed outside in one of the empty chairs surrounding the smoldering fire, listening to the oak crackle and spit out the end of its life. When she finally stood up to leave, she looked around at all the empty chairs, thanking the Lord for such a perfect day.

Betty no longer pleaded with Him to spare her child's life. She knew it was selfish and beyond His control, so she thanked Him for everything instead.

The same morning Charly died his new wife was in the Ottumwa hospital having a baby boy she named Jacob. A crazy guilt was felt by all who welcomed this child into their lives. Torn between the beginning of a new life and the end of a familiar one, Hugh and Betty couldn't or wouldn't leave their son, whose wishes were to die at home.

Eileen didn't want to leave her dying husband's bedside but was pried away by her parents when her labor pains grew too close and too strong. The sadness each of them felt for not being together was like an epidemic that lingered and consumed them over the many months that followed.

Charly was buried in the family graveyard on the hill near the river, a short walking distance from the house. He was with generations of his people, and now it was their job to look after the beautiful blue-eyed boy named Charly.

After he died, the three of them busied themselves with the new little boy. They tried desperately to replace their grief with the joy a baby is supposed to bring to a family but covering over the emptiness caused them to unknowingly poison each other by not dealing with their sadness and loss.

Hugh had hoped that this new boy, Jacob, could save his wife from herself, because her absentmindedness was a growing worry. In the meantime, Eileen—although attentive to her son—was void of any emotion, including the obvious attachment that one should have with their child. Concerned, Hugh called Eileen's parents and suggested they take her and the baby home with them for a while, which they eagerly did. It turned out to be a good place to heal and get attached. Slowly, Eileen morphed into the mother she had intended to be. Her devotion and love to her son was unbreakable.

Once a week their daughter-in-law brought Jacob out to the farm so Hugh and Betty could snuggle him and breathe in the air that escaped his little mouth. They were grateful to have Jacob and Eileen in their lives, but it was bittersweet watching him laugh and play and grow into a little version of Charly, then see them climb into their car and disappear for another week.

NOW

Hugh woke up the next morning with a crimp in his neck from sleeping in the chair all night. It was rare for him to sleep through the night, not to have gotten up at some point to go to the bedroom.

He stood up to stretch his old body, get his bearings, and shake the dream away. "Rise and shine everybody!" he said out of habit. Rubbing his stiff neck, he walked into the bedroom to wake his wife and found the bed was empty and the dresser drawer hung open. The bird was gone and so was Betty—again.

He called her name as he rushed through the house, running outside when he was unable to find her. Before he could check the back of the house to see if she was in the same place as the day before, he noticed Eileen's car coming up the driveway.

"Hugh what's wrong?" Eileen called, climbing out of the driver's seat. "Where's Betty?"

"I don't know," he managed to say, throwing his arms in the air before moving as fast as he could around the house.

Eileen and Jacob hurried after him, helping to shout for the old woman.

"Betty?"

"Grandma?"

The chorus of calling sounded throughout the yard.

The three of them ran in different directions around the farm. Hugh ran to the old barn while Eileen ran to stockyard. Jacob spotted her in the chicken coop gathering eggs. "Grandma, you okay?" he asked, feeling proud of himself for finding her first. He'd recently had his tenth birthday, and he was old enough to know about dementia. He didn't quite understand the disease, but he knew that his grandmother couldn't be left on her own. When he was sure she wasn't in any danger, he sprinted back out of the building, hollering, "She's in here, she's in here!"

Eileen came in first, relief relaxing her face, and Hugh was panting with beads of sweat glistening on his upper lip when he made it over.

"Good job, kiddo." Hugh praised Jacob with a pat on his shoulder while the three of them squeezed their way into the small coop.

Betty was using the front of her nightgown as a makeshift basket, and she had a collection of brown eggs nestled in the fabric. Under her feet and scattered around on the floor were Hugh's hankies.

Eileen backed out of the building, motioning for Jacob to follow. On her way past Hugh she whispered, "You okay?"

Hugh nodded, never taking his eyes off Betty.

"Jacob and I will go make some breakfast. You holler if you need anything." With a sad look on her face Eileen shut the creaky door behind them.

Hugh had known the day would come when he could no longer keep his wife safe. Standing there in the chicken coop, he feared that day had arrived.

"You scared me, woman," he said as he began transferring the eggs from her clothing to a nearby basket. "What am I to do, sweetheart?"

He wasn't expecting an answer and was a little surprised when Betty reached over and placed a hand on his arm. Then she pointed to a nearby nesting box where he was startled to see the forgotten bird. She gingerly touched the bird's little belly and said, "Breakfast."

The word and her actions made him smile, giving him reason to doubt the constant feeling of defeat. Even the fear he felt at finding her missing moments ago was replaced by amused relief and affection.

"Breakfast it will be," he said, setting the basket of eggs on a shelf and diving right into her world. It was something her doctor suggested he do rather than the impossible feat of trying to bring her bring her back into his. He played along with her by reaching into a bucket of scratch—feed reserved for young chicks—and holding out a handful to her so she might feed Boy.

She turned away from his hand, and for a fearful moment he could feel that glimmer of hope ebbing from his heart. Before it receded completely, he watched as her crooked fingers reached into the dirty windowsill and grabbed a clump of flies. He couldn't keep his mouth from dropping open as he watched her hold the insects in front of the bird. The scene reminded him of all the times she and Charly had nursed a critter of one kind or another. Hugh had lost count of all the animals they'd saved.

"Wife," Hugh said in a delicate tone after a few minutes passed, and the bird still hadn't responded. "I think he might be too far gone to eat." He was deliberating over how to go about leading her out of the coop when the bird stood up, nipped the flies from her fingers, and swallowed them up hungrily. The action seemed to wear the little guy out because soon afterward he fell backwards into the chicken box.

Hugh couldn't believe it. She did it, by God!

Tickled at her success, he waited to see what was next, satisfied when Betty turned towards the door and held out her arm for his.

"Now that the bird has eaten, I think it's our turn, don't you?" Hugh asked her with a wink. He couldn't be sure, but he thought he felt her give his arm a friendly squeeze as he led her inside.

BOY

Wife stole me out of the darkness and took me to a different place with wire screens and wooden slats—a smelly room where other prisoners are kept. She laid me down deep into one of the many humongous nests before she offered me food.

Once she left, I realized I couldn't see out of the nest. My only view was the occasional beady eyes that peeked over the box to check me out. Other prisoners of Old Man and Wife, I suspected. Normally, that would have scared me, but I was still so hungry that all I could focus on was the abundance of food flying lazily above my head, making my dry mouth water in anticipation. Easy pickins if I could only reach them.

I ignored all the curious eyes and put my energy into willing the flying morsels towards me. I'm pretty certain my leg is broken. When I managed to jump up to accept the "breakfast" Wife offered, a stinging pain ran from my leg and up into my head. I'm grateful it's only my leg and not my wings. A broken leg will heal, which means I'll need to be patient. When I'm stronger, I am gone, Johnson.

In the meantime, I'll find out if the other prisoners know the way out of here.

NEW DREAMS FOR OLD

There were four sitting at the table—five if you include Mrs. Nickels, who sat in Jacob's lap begging him with her eyes to share a bit of his scrambled eggs and toast with her.

Eileen volunteered to feed Betty her breakfast so Hugh could eat without interruption, while his food was still hot. The sheen in her eyes and the pitying tilt in her smile gave away the concern and worry Eileen felt for them. Hugh loved her for that. He loved her for so many reasons and being at their table right then was one of them.

Hugh wanted to tell Eileen about the past twenty-four hours, but he didn't know how to explain that the recent events, which included terrible fear and helplessness, also brought some small miracles.

Betty's mouth opened easily to the spoonful of egg that came her way. Hugh thought it ironic that she accepted food like a baby bird might do, opening her mouth wide after each bite, silently asking for more.

They watched as Betty slowly ate her food, never taking her eyes off Jacob. She was chewing far more than necessary, long after the food was gone from her mouth.

Jacob teased the cat with his own meal, and when Mrs. Nickels stole the toast right out of his hand and took off running, Betty laughed out loud. Soon everyone at the table was laughing with her.

When the meal was finished, Hugh led Betty to the familiar leather chair near the window. Jacob was right behind him, offering an afghan to cover Grandma's legs.

"Sweet boy," Hugh said as he ran his large hands through the boy's curly brown hair.

"Would you mind doing Grandpa a favor and feed the chickens?" he asked the boy. "It's worth a buck to ya."

"How about two bucks?" Jacob shot back.

"How about no bucks?" challenged his grandpa, beaming with a toothy grin.

"Okay Grandpa, a buck it is." And with that, Jacob turned and skipped out the door.

Eileen and Hugh stood next to each other at the kitchen sink, sharing in the dish duty. From the window, they watched the late morning sun beckon for Betty's eyes to close like clockwork.

Hugh was hungry to talk, but he didn't know where to begin, so he just started babbling like a man who'd been in solitary confinement.

He told her about the fear of losing his wife to the fields or to the road, and of course, to the nursing home. He talked about how the few chores he still had often went undone due to him not being able to leave Wife alone. This created his latest fear of not being able to keep up the farm. He heard his voice crack when he told her about the fits of anger and how Betty fought him like a stranger when he tried to bathe or clothe her. His cheeks were wet before he realized he was crying, and he brushed them with the dish towel, hoping Eileen wouldn't notice.

It seemed that many years' worth of sadness and fear poured out of him, but before he could get around to the good parts—the recent miracles—Eileen's heart could stand no more.

"Jacob and I want to move back to the farm," she blurted out.

Hugh could only blink at her at first. He had been waiting a long time to hear those words.

"I talked to Betty about it ages ago," Eileen explained. "I was waiting for you guys to give me the word, but that was before I realized the extent of the . . . memory issues. By then my own parents needed me, with their failing health and all. I felt so torn."

Hugh shuddered as she told him about her parent's recent decision to move into Silver Woods, an assisted living facility in Ottumwa. Fara Kremer and her brother financed the facility from the ground up, which was no small feat. Eileen's parents told her that they no longer wanted the responsibility of a home and all that comes with it. Her parents were excited by the idea of community living and eager for the many activities that were offered. The idea of that kind of living, Hugh could not fathom.

Hugh's eyebrows lifted in curious surprise.

"It was completely their choice," Eileen assured him. "They've always liked to do things their own way. It's a beautiful place, and they'll be well taken care of—medication, meals, doctor appointments, you name it. The responsibility of owning a home had just become too much for them, and they like the idea! You should see the activities the place offers!"

"You're sure they didn't . . ." Hugh wasn't sure how to phrase what was on his mind. "I mean, you didn't make them feel like they had to . . . for us?"

"No, no!" Eileen said. "To be honest, I begged them to stay at home! But this is what they wanted, Hugh."

He grabbed hold of her like she had just handed him the cure to everything sick and evil in the world and held her tight against his large chest. When he finally released her, he did so with an apology. "Honey, I'm sorry, but I can't ask you to give up the freedom your parents just gave back to you, only so you can return to the same isolation and responsibility. As much as we would love to have you here, I can't do that to you."

Eileen wouldn't have it. "This is what I want, it's what Jacob wants. This has always felt like our home. I wouldn't be giving up anything to come here, I'd be *home* again! I wanted nothing more than for my parents to stay in their own home, and I would've stayed with them until the very end and been okay with it, but believe it or not, they were bored, said they felt like the walls were closing in on them. Living in town isn't the same as living in the country, but you know that. Out here when you feel antsy there are options, like going outside." She laughed but kept going. "Jacob needs the farm like you need the farm, but most of all Hugh, he needs a man in his life, someone to teach him things I can't. I'm lucky that Charly's life insurance made it so I haven't had to worry about money—it's given me the freedom to be available to my son and my family in a way that I couldn't be if I were working—but even though Jacob has my time, it doesn't make up for not having a father. Please Hugh, let me share the freedom Charly left me with you and Betty."

Tears zigzagged through the untended whiskers on Hugh's face, but this time he didn't bother to wipe them away. He knew that she and Jacob were the answer to his prayers—a gift from God, or a gift from Charly. "Well, sugar, since you put it that way."

Seeing his approval, Eileen raced ahead with her speech. "If it's okay, we could move in by the end of the week. I already have a renter for mom and dad's house. I was thinking I could visit them at the facility in the mornings after I drop Jacob off at school. And he could ride home on the bus, so I don't have to make both trips." She'd thought this through ahead of time, and the genuine excitement radiating off her was contagious. "It's a deal then?" she asked, sticking out her hand.

"It's a deal," he agreed, shaking her hand in such an exaggerated way that it made them both smile.

"I'll go tell Jacob the good news!" she said, heading outside. But first, she turned around and said, "Thank you, Hugh, from the bottom of my heart."

Hugh watched from the window as Eileen headed for the chicken coop. "No, thank *you*," he whispered.

BOY MEETS BOY

Jacob was sitting on a shelf, squeezed in between the nesting boxes, when his mom came into the coop. The building was empty except for Jacob and Mrs. Nickels, who sat on the floor watching him.

"What's up bud?" Eileen asked, walking over to where her son sat. "I thought you'd be outside feeding the chickens."

"I already fed them," he said. "Come here and look at this, mom."

Eileen moved in close, following her son's eyes to one of the boxes. Inside, a little bird was staring up at them—a sparrow of some kind she guessed.

"What the heck?" she whispered.

"I tried to stand him up, but he keeps falling over," Jacob said with concern. "I think he's broken."

"Well then," Eileen said softly. "Let's leave him alone and let nature take its course, honey."

"But we can't just leave him out here to die," Jacob pleaded. "Can't I at least try to feed him?"

Eileen appeared to consider that. "You can try, but I wouldn't touch him any more than you have to. You don't want to give the little guy a heart attack before he has the chance to heal."

Eileen sat down on a wooden crate before realizing the fresh gob of chicken poop on top of it that was now stuck to her clothes. "Dang it," she mumbled. She watched her son successfully feed a bug to the bird. Then he took a water bottle from his pocket, dribbled some onto his fingers, and let the drops fall onto the bird's beak.

"You are your father's son, that's for sure," she said as she stood up and rubbed her butt along the rough wooden planks of the wall, removing some of the poop from the seat of her pants. "When you're done playing doctor, why don't you clean out the coop for Grandpa? I'm sure he would appreciate it." Then before Jacob could protest, she added, "As a matter of fact, this can be one of your daily chores from now on—now that we're going to be living here!"

Jacob clapped his hands, hopping up to grab hold of his mom, when his jacket snagged the corner of the nesting box, turning it upside down and tumbling it to the ground.

It happened so fast that neither of them could catch the box before it landed, spilling its contents and the little bird inside onto the damp floor. Before they could pick up the injured bird, Mrs. Nickels snatched it up in her mouth and ran out the coop door. As if making a delivery, she dropped the bird in the middle of the pen. Out of nowhere came a massive rooster who quickly sat on the poor thing.

"Shit!" Jacob screamed in horror.

"What did you just say?" Eileen's voice went up an octave.

"I meant 'shoot,' mom. Now what are we supposed to do?" he cried.

Eileen decided the time for expert intervention had come. "I have a feeling Grandpa knows a little something about this bird, so why don't you go ask him to come on out here?"

Sensing the commotion in the yard, Betty scooted her way out of the chair, and by the time Hugh reached her, she was standing. "Boy," she said, pointing to the kitchen door.

Jacob burst through the door, panting the words, "Grandpa, you gotta come help!"

Hugh steadied his wife and said, "Well, let's go see what's going on out there."

When the old couple arrived on the scene, Eileen and Jacob were surrounded by pecking chickens and one stubborn, immovable rooster.

"Grandpa," Jacob said breathlessly, pointing. "That old rooster is sitting on a little bird, and the hens won't let us get near it! It's going to get smothered if we don't do something quick!"

"Is that so?" Hugh asked. Then he stepped in closer to the gang of noisy chickens as Betty squeezed his arm so hard it hurt.

"Boy," she said pointing to the rooster.

Hugh reached over and patted the top of Jacob's head. "Yep, boy," he said to his wife.

Betty shook her head angrily. "No!" She freed herself from his grip, and with little effort, bent down and gently pushed the rooster aside, exposing the little bird with big black eyes. She picked it up with cupped hands and, without a second's hesitation, headed back into the coop.

Eileen searched Hugh's face for an explanation, but all he could do was catch up with his wife. "I'll explain later," he said. "If I can." The creaky coop door closed behind him.

Betty had already put the tiny bird back in a nesting box when Hugh came in behind her. He'd be damned if he could understand her fascination with this bird, but he had to admit that it was a pleasant distraction from the gloom filling most of their time together of late.

"Boy?" he asked cautiously, deciding to go back into her world. That bird was the only thing that seemed to be consistent in her mixed-up mind these days.

In a flash, she turned to face him, wearing an impish smile and a light in her eyes that said, "Yes, you dummy!" She turned back around and gently patted the little bird on its head.

After a few minutes, she turned again, but this time it was because she could tell he was ready to leave. "House," she instructed, holding out her arm to her husband.

"Whatever you say, woman," he replied gallantly, and for the second time that day, he guided her out of the coop and back into the house.

When they came through the door, Eileen and Jacob were back at the table waiting for them. Hugh held up his hand as if to say "later," then helped Betty into a chair across from them and sat close to her. He looked across the table and grinned—he couldn't help it. He hadn't felt this good in an exceedingly long time.

"You know what I think, Jacob?" Hugh asked. "I think it's time we get you an animal or two to look after. Maybe something you can take to the fair come next summer. How's that sound to you?"

Jacob stood up so fast he knocked over his chair. "Really, Grandpa, really? An animal of my own? Mom, did you hear that?"

Before Eileen could say anything, Betty started clapping. The cheer spread over everyone like rising sunshine and they all joined in. When they realized that Betty had stopped—hunched shoulders and distant eyes—their own clapping faded into silence. The celebration had ended almost as fast as it started, but it had been a great one, nonetheless.

BOY

This is going to sound weak, like I'm backpedaling from my original plan, but for the record, I want to say that I'm no longer afraid for my life. I no longer fear that I'm in the hands of the enemy—other than, of course, the furry one, who the jury's still out on.

It did grab me in its mouth, but it didn't hurt me, which it certainly could have. Instead, it took me away to safety, to another prisoner who hid me underneath his own body, reminding me of my mother and how she kept me safe and warm.

I miss my mother and wonder where she might be.

Don't get me wrong: I still plan on leaving when I'm able, but now that I feel protected, I can be more patient. Food is available and so is the large nest that I wish I could see out of. The only other thing I wish for is someone to talk to, someone like me.

THE POWER OF LOVE AND MEMORY

After a late lunch, Eileen informed Hugh that she and Betty were going to clean out the bedrooms to get them ready for the big move-in on Friday, and suggested the guys find something to do outside.

"Are you sure you don't want two big strapping men to help you move things around?" Hugh asked.

Jacob laughed, flexing his own arm, and checking for any new muscle growth. He was more enthusiastic about getting outside than proving his strength, though. Relief was written all over his face when his mom refused the offer.

"No, but thanks anyway. I think we can manage without you, can't we, Betty?"

Betty stood alone, looking out the kitchen window. She didn't respond or even glance at them, not that anyone really expected her to. Including her in conversation was done out of courtesy and habit. She had always been an important part of their lives, so why should that change now that she had an illness? It was something none of them would ever quit doing. She was a part of their world even if they were strangers to her.

Eileen scooted the guys out the door, then gently took Betty's arm and led her to the bed in Charly's old room. She perched on the edge like a statue, watching every move Eileen made—uninterested or unaware that she was surrounded in the leavings of her son's young life.

"This will be Jacob's room," Eileen announced, while removing the contents of the closet. She boxed everything away, purposely not pausing over the soft cotton t-shirts and sturdy button-downs her husband once wore. She would save those reflections for another day when she could handle seeing the things that represented the man she could no longer hold or deal with the irony of his mother's fading memories, already boxed and sealed away, forever.

By the time she finished the closet and moved on to the dresser, Betty had fallen asleep. Still sitting upright on the bed, she looked like a rag doll, leaning precariously to one side, ready to fall over any minute. Eileen eased her down and spread a blanket over her little body that once covered Charly. It no longer smelled of the man she knew but of must and dust and years of being ignored by a washing machine.

Next, she emptied the drawers of old clothes and various rocks that once had significance and put them in one of the many boxes at her feet. She saved out the arrowheads she ran across for Jacob's growing collection. She came upon a photo she couldn't ignore, much less pack away. In it was a tall, gangly boy standing next to a cow that wore a big blue ribbon around its neck. The inscription told her that it was taken in 1990 at the Wapello County Fair. A proud teenage boy stood with his hand on top of one of his prized animals. As she studied the photo a voice behind her said, "Daisy."

Startled, she turned around to find Betty standing so close that it gave her goose bumps. She was looking at the photo as intently as Eileen.

Once Eileen's heart went back to its normal rhythm, she led Betty back to the bed, where they both sat down.

"Daisy," Betty said again, not taking her eyes off the photo.

Pointing to Charly, Eileen asked, "Who's that standing next to Daisy?"

A little laugh escaped Betty's mouth. "Boy," she answered.

Hoping her cognizant state would continue, Eileen handed the photo to Betty and went back to the dresser and dug around until she found more photos of Charly. There were ones of him riding a horse, playing baseball, and one of him standing next to a dozen other boys who all wore Boy Scout uniforms. She returned to the bed and displayed the photos in her hand like a fan.

"Who's this?" she asked, pointing to Charly in each photo.

"Boy, boy, boy," Betty said, tapping each photo with determination.

"Yes, your *boy!*" Eileen repeated excitedly. She tried to prompt the older woman into sharing more about the photos, but it wasn't to be. However, before fading completely away, she reached over and took the photos out of Eileen's hand, forcing them into the small pocket of her dress, crinkling and tearing them until succeeding. Then she lay back down on her son's bed and closed her eyes.

At first, Eileen thought Betty was closing her eyes to shut out the painful memories that flooded the now empty room, but when she began to snore, Eileen realized that the moment to reflect had simply come and gone. There was no deep meaning or reasoning to any of it—which was disappointing no matter how many times it happened.

Eileen knew dementia was unpredictable, like a train that runs on and off its tracks, out of control and with no one driving it. Even so, she couldn't wait to share this interlude with Hugh. She couldn't wait to help connect the dots that led from Charly to the bird Betty called "Boy."

By the time Hugh and Jacob returned to the house they were filthy and sweaty. They were talking about their great new plan as they came into the kitchen, and as soon as Jacob saw his mother, he began rattling off all they had accomplished in the barn.

"Slow down kid, so I can understand you," Eileen said.

It was apparent looking at Hugh how much he needed days like this one. His happiness was evident from his smiling face down to his dirty boots.

"We cleaned out the stalls to get them ready for my animals—I mean our animals," the boy gushed, smiling at his Grandpa. "First, we're going to get a cow, then maybe a pig or two, but first we're going to get a cow. And I'm going to name it Daisy, right Grandpa?"

When Eileen heard the name Daisy, she almost fell over. Hugh went over to where she stood and took her hand. "Are you okay honey?" he asked. "You look like you just saw a ghost?"

"I think maybe I have," she whispered under her breath.

"Woman, you look a bit pale. I think you wore yourself clean out. How about you call it quits for the day while Jacob and I make some tea?" Not waiting for an answer, he added, "Where's Betty?"

Hanging onto the counter with one hand she answered, "She's in Charly's room, sleeping."

It wasn't that he didn't trust Eileen—he trusted her with his life—but he also knew that his wife hadn't been in Charly's room for years. Neither of them had.

Hugh left her side and walked straight to Charly's bedroom where he hesitated in the doorway. From there he saw Betty on the bed, asleep. He looked around, taking in the emptiness and the boxes scattered on the floor. After a few minutes, he backed out and went to sit at the table.

Eileen hadn't thought about how he would feel about the changes she'd made in Charly's room. "I'm sorry, Hugh. I guess I wasn't thinking. I'm such a schmuck."

Hugh held up his hand and said, "You're no schmuck, it's just a shock. You would think after all this time we would be over it. To be honest with you honey, neither of us have stepped foot in there in years and that's certainly not your fault."

Eileen walked over and put her arms around Hugh's neck, hugging his head and shoulders. "We'll get through this together, I promise you that. Now how about a cup of tea? You look like you could use it more than I can."

Hugh was smiling at her when Jacob piped up, "What in the hell is wrong with everybody? I haven't even got to finish telling you our plans."

Eileen's nostrils flared and her eyes widened. "It's going to be awful hard for you to tell us with a bar of soap stuffed in your mouth, young man!"

Jacob shrunk in on himself, withdrawing as his mother came near. "Whoops . . ." he said, backing into the refrigerator as he retreated. "I'm sorry, it just slipped out!" He looked beseechingly to his Grandpa to save him.

"Yes, it would be a good time for tea about now, don't you agree son?" Hugh asked, trying to hold back the laugh that wanted to escape his mouth.

"I sure do, Grandpa, and I'll even make it for you guys. Mom, go sit down and hug Grandpa some more while I make your tea."

That cracked up Hugh and Eileen couldn't hide her amusement either.

"He just saved himself from talking with bubbles for the next couple hours," she said before joining him in a good laugh at the table.

After tea and conversation about which animals they should get first, Eileen got up to warm the supper she'd brought. Hugh thought he'd died and gone to heaven as he ate the hamburger gravy, mashed potatoes, and home-canned peaches for dessert.

Betty slept through it all. Hugh kept checking on her, making sure she hadn't slipped out the window or a crack somehow. He watched closely to make sure her chest was rising and falling in rhythm.If she were too quiet or still, he'd put his cheek near her lips to feel for that whisper of breath. His fear of losing her was so great that even as she slept his nerves were on edge.

His concern was obvious to Eileen, and she was happy that soon she could help him full time. *Soon*, she thought, *we'll take shifts, and the old man will be able to take care of himself for a change*.

She wanted to tell him about the photos and how Betty identified Charly in all of them. She wanted to tell him about Daisy the cow and the coincidence from earlier in the day, but Hugh looked tired and preoccupied. Heck, she was tired and preoccupied with her own thoughts as well.

Deciding it could all wait for another day; they said their goodbyes. Jacob fell fast asleep as they drove away from the farm. The fresh air tuckered him out, which she believed was the best medicine . . . for anyone.

Eileen watched the sun disappear from the sky as she made the last corner to her house. Pulling up in front of it, she parked but didn't get out. Her eyes drifted over the old home as her son slept in the back seat. She studied the small yard and remembered the many games of tag played in it. She looked at the porch with its glowing overhead light and saw the familiar, mysterious shadows reflected in the windows—the ones that always scared her as a child. Just beyond the fence, alongside the cottonwood tree, stood the playhouse that was once the neighborhood hangout. It was also Eileen's refuge when she needed to disappear.

She knew she could walk away from all of it and not feel guilty or sad because her parents had done it. They left to begin a new life for themselves while the choice was still theirs, and Eileen was excited to do the same for herself and her son.

"We're excited for something new," Eileen's dad, Bob, had said as he finished loading up their van on moving day.

Her mom, Kathy, was so giddy that she buckled herself in the passenger seat long before her husband had finished packing everything up. When her dad slid the door shut for the last time, her mother hung out the window and said to Eileen, "Don't be sad honey, it's just a house. Our memories aren't inside those walls. Our memories are inside us." She handed over their house keys and, with a wave, added, "We'll see you guys soon, once we get settled in honey."

Eileen had watched as the loaded down van drove away, her parents all smiles like they were going on some exotic vacation. Their words had given her the permission she needed to do the same—to move on.

She looked away from her childhood home and up to the Big Dipper. As she got out of the car, she said, "Thanks mom and dad." Then she roused her son awake.

THE IMPORTANCE OF PURPOSE

The next day was much like the ones before, except that Hugh woke with a purpose that fueled him. Soon the chairs around the table would be filled on a regular basis. Chatter and the smell of good food would bless the old, quiet rooms. These were little things that he had missed terribly but hadn't realized just how much until right then.

He was excited at the thought of returning to the projects and chores he once enjoyed, thanks to Eileen. Just thinking about cleaning out the garden for next spring's planting made his mouth water for fresh peas and tomatoes.

Soon he would have uninterrupted time to spend with his grandson. He would teach him about the farm, and everything involved in making it work. But most importantly, he knew that his old house would feel like a home again, and that realization filled him with joy and anticipation.

With breakfast over and Betty asleep in the chair, he decided that it was time to tackle the clutter on the table he'd ignored for so long. He would make room for the ones who would soon be occupying it. By the time he finished sorting through the piles of paper, he was surprised that most of it was just junk, leaving little to even file away. Something that took years to accumulate took only minutes to throw away. "Imagine that," he mumbled.

He stood and looked at the empty table. Now it was too bare, so he went to the buffet against the wall between the living room and kitchen, searching through drawers until he found the most colorful doily. He placed it in the middle of the table, giving it some color and little life. But it still wasn't enough, so he added the salt and pepper shakers and stood back to admire his work when Betty woke up with a whimper.

Helping her up from the chair, he found that she was soaking wet, her dress clinging to her spindly legs. *No wonder she woke up*, he thought to himself. "Poor baby, let's get you cleaned up and then we'll go feed the chickens."

She didn't look at him, staring at something faraway. Today that didn't grab at his heart the way it usually did. He was slowly accepting that she lived in some other place, and he knew that he was lucky she was here at all.

In the bedroom, he peeled away her drenched clothes and cleaned her legs and private area with a warm washcloth—his hands moving apprehensively as he tested how she would receive his touch. As he dabbed away the urine from her pale skin, she began to hum. Relieved that she was no longer whimpering, and thrilled that she wasn't fighting him, he tried in vain to place the familiar tune.

After buttoning up a clean dress for her, he tossed the wet clothes into the nearby laundry basket, and something caught his eye. He reached down to remove several squares of thick, glossy paper from the pocket of the dress his wife had worn the day before, and when he'd succeeded, blood rushed to his face, making him feel lightheaded. He sat down on the bed next to Betty and stared at the face that seemed to stare back at him.

He studied each picture, smoothing the torn edges and creases with care, remembering the day each and every one was taken. He'd never realized how much his grandson looked like his Charly. It was the first time he could look at his son and not be consumed with grief.

Hugh had been lost in memories for so long he'd almost forgotten his wife sitting quietly beside him. "How about we go see how your feathered friend is today?" he asked her. "I bet he's one hungry Boy."

The magic word had been spoken. Betty turned toward her husband, head cocked, the cloudy look in her eyes parting as they focused. She slowly took the photos from his loose grasp. "Boy," she said, pointing to their son.

"Oh my God," Hugh muttered, connecting the dots. "Let's go feed that Boy, woman!" He was filled with a powerful energy, the familiar despair that walked alongside him for so many months was nowhere to be found. He wouldn't question it and he sure wasn't going to go looking for it. It would find him soon enough. Of that he was certain.

THE BIRD WHISPERER

Clouds filled the sky as they made their way to the chicken coop. Leaves danced in their path and circled the mob of hungry chickens. Soon the snow would come and cover everything in a blanket of white. He knew that if he was going to get Jacob some critters, he'd better get on it.

After supper he would call his neighbor Fara and see if they couldn't do a trade for a young cow or two. He knew she could use the hay in his lower field, and with the weather permitting there was still time for her brothers to mow and harvest it.

He smiled when he realized that with animals on their way, he could use some hay this winter himself. Just thinking about that filled his nostrils with the sweet earthy scent.

Once they cleared the doorway, he released her arm so she could walk alone to her nesting Boy. Hugh left her alone in the coop while he fed the chickens in the open pen. There was no fear of her escaping without going past him first. The worst thing he figured could happen was that she would forget why she was in there.

When he was finished, he joined her inside, pleased to find her sitting on the lower shelf, squeezed in between two boxes, and holding the bird in the palm of her hand. She was humming the same tune that she had before, but just when he had the name of the tune on the tip of his tongue, the bird startled him by flying onto one of the windowsills.

Betty started to stand, and Hugh instinctively held out his arm to stop her. He pushed an empty box out of his way with his other hand so he could sit next to her on the shelf. They sat scrunched together like sardines in a can, watching the bird pluck imprisoned flies from the windowsill, Betty giggling in delight.

She turned to him, and he thought back to the many high school football games they went to—first at their own school and then Charly's—scrunched together on cold bleachers like they were now, happily keeping each other warm.

Her breath on his neck broke his trance as she said the same word as before, but with pride. "Boy." It was the same pride she had so many years ago when Charly scored a touchdown or ran the ball down the field with those stocky legs of his, dodging his opponents.

He watched her turn back towards the window and the bird. He was so happy, yet so afraid at the same time. Even in the depths of her dementia she had insisted on saving this little bird from death, and she had succeeded.

He was in awe that a bird, a simple little bird, could stir up her tangled and dying memories when nothing else had—not medication, family, friends, or even her husband of many decades. There was no way to explain it, not to anyone.

Selfishly, he worried that now that the mystery of the bird was over, so might be the joy it had brought to their lives. Now that it could fly away, surely it would do just that.

Hugh waited at least fifteen minutes before he stood up to leave, silently telling himself that what will be, will be.

He held out his hand to support Betty as she stepped down safely, and the bird flew out of the windowsill and landed on her shoulder! Hugh stared in disbelief; Betty only chuckled more as the three of them walked out into the cloud-covered morning. The bird teetered on her bony shoulder, clinging with its little feet to her dress. The chickens ignored them as they passed.

As a test, Hugh walked them towards the barn, just to see how long it would take before the bird released its grip and flew away. It didn't take long. As soon as they cleared the barn doors, the bird released the hold it had on the thin cotton dress and flew to a nearby rafter. When their eyes adjusted to the natural light inside the barn, Hugh pointed to the bird perched on one of the large timbers, looking down at them.

Out of nowhere, Mrs. Nickels appeared at their feet, taking in the action too, until a mouse ran across the dirt floor. Then, as fast as her legs would take her, she was off.

Hugh knew this was it. For the first time since her disease took everything familiar away from her, he found himself praying that she would forget the bird, just so she wouldn't be let down by its departure.

As a distraction, he guided her to the newly clean stalls, explaining—unnecessarily and to fill a void—that soon Jacob's calves would be living there.

"Daisy?" she asked, leaning on the wooden boards that separated the stalls.

"No. I mean yes! Daisy will be here and so will Bob and Lord knows who else," he said with a chuckle.

"Boy?" She asked with searching eyes.

"I don't know, Wife. Maybe. Boy has to go home sometime. His mama must be missing him something terrible, don't you think?" he replied, reaching for anything to satisfy her obsession.

She put her hands on her chest and said, "Mama." That single word broke his heart, but he wasn't going to let it break his spirit.

"Yes, you are a mama, and a very good one at that," he added, covering her tiny hands with his own large ones. He would do and say anything that calmed her, even if it meant lying or, Lord knows, finding her another bird to focus on.

The little bird was the apparent substitute for the son she no longer had. At least that's the conclusion the dots had led him to.

They had almost reached the house when the wind arrived, blowing dust and loose leaves around at Mach speed, creating a sound he'd loved since childhood.

He noticed the chickens heading for the opening in the coop, seeking shelter from the wind as fast as they could. "Smart," Hugh said and shielded his eyes as he hurried Betty towards the kitchen door.

Before they took the last few steps to the door, he saw something move out of the corner of his eye. At first, he thought it was a shingle on the chicken coop flapping in the wind, but then he saw it was a bird that looked very much like the one they'd left in the barn. It stood on the edge of the coop's roof, fighting the wind, and watching the chickens scramble in through the hole in the building.

Impossible, he thought. *It's just a sparrow*. There must be millions of birds in Iowa that looked just like this one. But why was it out in the weather when all the other birds had sought shelter? This was either a coincidence, or he was losing his mind.

"How can this be?" he said into the side of his wife's head. "You're the bird whisperer, what do you think?"

Her head was turned down, avoiding the wind. He didn't expect an answer, nor did he get one. It was partly out of habit that he'd asked.

Curiosity had gotten the best of him. He had to go check out this bird, and he had to take Betty along with him. There would be no more leaving her out of his sight, at least not until Eileen was there.

"Would you look at that, woman? Your Boy wants back in his house!"

She'd been mesmerized by a button on her dress when she heard the magic word. Her head jerked up to the sky, searching . . . searching.

"Over there," Hugh said, pointing to the strange little bird that stood on its edge, defying the strong wind.

Betty immediately pulled away from him and headed towards the bird, when the darn thing swooped down and met her halfway, landing on her shoulder, again!

The hair on Hugh's arms stood up as he caught up to her, taking her arm as they neared the coop. As soon as he opened the door, the bird left her shoulder, flew in, and landed on the side of the same box it had inhabited for two days. But a chicken had already beaten him to the nest.

Betty didn't appear phased at all by what had just happened, nor did she want to linger. She simply reached over and pulled the string on the wall-mounted light bulb (meant to radiate warmth on cold days). Then, when she turned to go, she whispered, "Nighty, night."

THE GIFT OF HUMOR

By the time they cleared the doorway, a cold rain had started, sending shivers up Hugh's spine, matching the sensation of the goosebumps that still covered his arms. He walked into the warm kitchen and filled the tea kettle with water, putting it on the stove to heat. Before he took the cups to the table he reached inside the overhead cupboard and grabbed the bottle of brandy he kept for "times of need." As he dumped a shot in with his tea, he concluded this was definitely one of those times.

The brandy burned as it slid down into his belly. It felt good—too good. Knowing he shouldn't have anymore, he got up, went back into the kitchen, and made them a couple grilled cheese sandwiches which were also pretty darn good.

In between bites, Betty fiddled with the buttons on her dress while her gaze was fixed on the far end of the table where the old photos of Charly rested. Releasing the hold on her buttons, her hands reached across the table and slid the photos in front of Hugh. He looked down at them, then back to her. She smiled, and that's when he decided he was no longer going to be afraid of whatever ride they were on. Instead, he was going to ride it hard, right up until the end of time.

Outside, the wind banged the old shutters ruthlessly against the side of the house. After dinner, Hugh helped Betty into the leather chair near the window where they watched a variety of small items fly by, reminiscent of the tornado scenes in *The Wizard of Oz*.

It had been years since a tornado touched down in their county, and many years more since the farm was hit by one. The memory of missing livestock and splintered debris added to the chill he felt, so he turned the heat on for the first time that fall. By the time he was back from the thermostat, she was asleep. *Full tummies do that to a person*, he thought.

He knew he couldn't afford to fall asleep yet in case Betty should wake. The risk wasn't worth it, so instead he busied himself with the sign he was making for Jacob. It was for the barn and would read "Jacob's Farm" in big black letters. He would hang it next to the faded one with "Charly's Farm" painted on. Maybe one day Jacob would make his own sign with his child's name on it, adding it to the barn. The thought was as warm as the brandy.

He'd just finished painting the last letter on the sign when the phone began to ring, startling him. He hurried into the kitchen, grabbing a paper towel to wipe paint off his hands, but before he could get to the phone, the ringing had stopped, and he heard Betty say, "Hello?"

With all the strange happenings lately, he shouldn't have been surprised that she'd answered the phone. *Anything's possible*, he thought as he walked back into the room. He burst into laughter, though, when he saw that she hadn't picked up the phone at all, but a statue of Roy Rogers that sat next to her on the end table. She was holding it up against her ear, as if waiting for someone to answer her greeting.

Hugh couldn't help himself. "Who is it?" he asked.

Sitting Roy back down on the table, she said, "They hung up."

"They'll call back," Hugh said, laughing so hard his stomach ached. And they did call back, but by then Betty was no longer interested. She had faded away again.

It was Eileen calling to check in and to let him know that Saturday was the big day. "I'm just taking a break before packing up the rest of my parent's things," she said, fatigue dragging down some of the pumped-up excitement in her tone. "Jacob and I spent the evening packing up our things, so at least that's all finished."

Hugh couldn't help it, walking into the other room and quietly sharing with Eileen what had just happened when Betty tried to answer the phone. When she cracked up laughing, he was relieved that she didn't judge him for finding humor in his wife's confusion.

To have a little humor, and to have it without feeling guilt, is a blessing, he thought as he returned the phone to the table, next to Roy.

That night, as he lay down next to Betty, he thought of the big days ahead. Only two more before Jacob and Eileen would be moved in.

He kicked himself for not remembering to tell Eileen that Fara would be delivering the calves that day too. He was so excited that he didn't think he would ever fall asleep, but soon his mind settled, and his old, worn-out body finally relented.

BOY

I was sure I would be stuck in that big old building for the night. Thank goodness for the cracks in the loft. They gave me options for escaping that scary place. I wouldn't have slept a wink with all the noises and bats flying around my head.

It's much warmer in here and much safer too. Now that I knew I wasn't a prisoner, and that the ones who shared these nests with me weren't being held against their will, I could relax a little and get some much-needed sleep.

My leg was still hurting. I felt a burning each time I took off. I think I just needed a little more time.

To be honest, I wasn't looking forward to finding a place to hole up for the winter. With any luck, Old Man and Wife wouldn't make me leave until I was ready. I'd guess that by spring my leg should be good as new.

Then all I had to do was just get the fatso in my nest to move over a little.

"Come on . . . scoot over, big mama," I encouraged, nudging her with my wing.

Once she moved over, it was perfect. What was it Wife said before she left? "Nighty, night?"

FRIENDSHIP

By the time Saturday rolled around, Hugh was eager for big changes. He was ready for Eileen and Jacob to call this home, ready for the smell and sounds of animals to surround him, ready for some new life and all the commotion it brings with it.

Hugh was just plain ready.

Fara told him that her spring calves were a gift, and so was the hay her brothers would deliver with the animals. "They'll be no arguing with me, Hugh. We're also going to cut your fields, so you don't have to worry about 'em going to waste. Maybe next year you can teach that boy of yours how to run a tractor," she insisted. Just the thought of that excited him to no end.

"How can I thank you, Fara?" he said, watching Betty sip her tea at the table.

"I'm just so happy that Eileen and Jacob are moving to the farm. I'm relieved to know you won't be alone this winter with Betty. It's way too big a job for one person. So please, there's no need to thank me, buddy."

"Well thank you anyway. I mean it," he said, raw emotion in his voice.

They'd been friends as well as neighbors since they were children, and they'd both experienced a lot of good and bad times in their life. That's always the story if you're lucky enough to live to old age. It's also one of the things that bind people together. Struggles, and surviving them, is what fills the pages of our history books. It's also what makes a friend a true one.

By the time breakfast was over, Hugh could hardly contain himself. The anticipation was driving him nuts. Deciding to put the dishes off until later, he put on his worn out Carhart jacket, and when he approached Betty with a sweater, she was lost in the wallpaper world, humming that same tune.

He sat down next to her and began putting her arms in the sleeves of the sweater when she started to scream. He tried to hold her, and the screaming grew louder, scaring the daylights out of him.

"No, no, no!" she screamed towards the wall.

He scooted a few inches away to give them both some room, then very softly said, "Shhhhh, it's okay, baby. Shhhhhh, it's okay." He said it over and over until her screaming eased to a whimper.

Eventually she turned to face him and said, "I want my mommy!"

This was new.

"Well love, she's not here right now," was all he could quickly come up with. It slowed the whimpering and ended her fascination with the wallpaper.

Cocking her head to one side, she asked, "Where's my mommy?"

"She's in town running errands, but she'll be back later," he improvised. "She said that we're supposed to do some chores around here before she gets back."

There were a few moments of silence. Then a little, "Okay," escaped her lips, and she began putting on her sweater all by herself.

Hugh felt a sudden wave of nausea. Between the excitement of what the day was to bring, and his wife's new confusion, he knew he needed to get a grip or risk ruining everything. He needed to preoccupy himself with something.

The chores. He'd do the chores.

They were walking through the kitchen towards the door when he remembered the mysterious bird and how it had appeared to want to be in the coop with the chickens. Impulsively, he grabbed the drill out of the closet. Maybe he could make a few improvements to the coop for the little guy and drill a few holes for coming and going. Maybe even put up a perch or two.

Once they cleared the few steps and were safely on the ground, he glanced over at Betty. He was relieved to see the calm on her face. Whatever it was that had made her scream bloody murder was forgotten, at least for the present.

The only good thing about the disease that ate away at her brain was that it worked like a slide show, presenting a fleeting image before quickly changing to another. Even if there were times he wanted the slide show to slow down, he was often grateful, for her sake, that it didn't.

For the first time, he wondered what stage she was in. He knew there were different stages to dementia, but he'd never looked them up, or asked the doctor about them. It was like he'd been living in a fog ever since she got sick. Only dealing on a surface level with what came his way, without any knowledge of what it meant or what was to come.

As the sun warmed his face, one thought was extremely clear: he could no longer predict what world she was living in at any given time. Her asking the whereabouts of her mother, who had been dead for decades, made him feel sad for the woman who shuffled along beside him—and especially sad for the little girl inside of her who missed her mommy.

As they made their way to the coop, he thought of his own parents and how long they'd been gone from his life. It's funny how no matter how old a person gets, they never quit missing their parents.

All of it made him think about the God he was raised to believe in, and he wondered why such a powerful being would allow such torture of the good and the innocent. None of it made any sense to him, and although he'd already decided that he was on this ride until the end, he prayed to the unfair God above to help him continue to find the right words to comfort her while on that journey.

A short, round woman with a dirty-brown bob emerged from the chicken coop with a basket of eggs, just as Hugh and Betty were approaching. "Oh!" she said, startled, surprising her as well as them.

Typically, Eliza—a church friend and local volunteer—collected the eggs for the food shelf early in the morning, before anyone at the farm was up and moving. Hugh often wondered if that was because of her busy schedule or if her timing was meant to avoid the uncomfortable conversations they had about Betty at times. Either way, it was fine by him.

Eliza was a few years behind Betty and Hugh in school, and even then, she was a pest, following them wherever they went. At age sixty-eight she wasn't much different, still poking into their business with her chubby, red cheeks—a clue to her high blood pressure. The only real difference today were the random specks of gray in her otherwise unchanging hairstyle.

Hugh and Betty would agree that she was a good woman, one who would do anything for anyone . . . except shut up when you needed her to. She volunteered at church, the food shelf, and prepared lunch seven days a week at the soup kitchen in downtown Ottumwa—all out of the goodness in her heart. Along with her "do-good" attitude, she was a bossy and opinionated woman, one lucky enough to catch a decent husband.

Hugh's biggest problem with Eliza was that she made it clear every chance she got how strongly she felt that Betty should be in a nursing home. When she told him that he couldn't possibly care for her the way she needed to be cared for, it hurt him, and he resented it deeply.

Eliza didn't understand that the farm was the one thing Betty still knew, and he wasn't about to take that away from her. He knew that moving her to an unfamiliar place would be the end of what was left of her, and as long as he was alive, that was not going to happen. No matter what anyone thought.

The subject of how to deal with Betty's deterioration was one Eliza brought up no matter where they happened to run into each other—grocery store, post office, pharmacy, or church—which is the biggest reason he avoided taking Betty into town. The sympathy and judgment he detected only made things harder on him.

The conversation was always the same, and inevitably both walked away frustrated.

She just didn't get his view of things and wouldn't shut up about it. He no longer had the energy to debate the issue with her, which is why they were both better off not having these forced conversations. It somehow took something real away from the hundreds, if not thousands, of great talks they'd had over the years.

"Hi, Hugh," Eliza said, looking Betty over while she set the basket of eggs on the hood of her car. "Hey, Betty, how you doing, honey?"

"Mom says we have to do our chores before she gets home," Betty responded to the greeting.

Eliza's curious expression twisted into ugly horror. *Here we go again*, Hugh thought to himself.

"Oh my God, Hugh, are you all right? Is everything here all right?" Eliza said, wiping her hands on her pants, but never taking her eyes off Betty.

Hugh noticed, as she continued her campaign to save the world, that her red lipstick was smeared all over her top teeth. It distracted him briefly, which was kind of nice. He chuckled inwardly at his private joke, but answered, "Yes Eliza, everything here is just peachy. How's everything with you?"

Eliza nervously ran her tongue over her teeth, as if sensing his private joke. "Fine," she managed to get out. "How's Betty, though? I mean, how is she, really?"

Hugh sighed heavily. "Eliza, you know my wife isn't well. That hasn't changed, but other than that she's fine, really." He tried not to sound as exasperated as he felt, changing the subject. "Today's a big day for us, isn't it dear?" He hugged Betty around the shoulders, giving her a bright smile. "Eileen and Jacob are moving to the farm and we have a lot to do to get ready, so if you'll excuse us?" Done with Eliza, he led Betty towards the barn.

"I heard they were moving in," Eliza said to his backside. "I'm real happy to hear that, Hugh, happy for all of you." She poured her round body into her car, but before she drove away, she rolled down the window and hollered, "By the way, there's an ugly little bird trapped in the coop with your chickens. It's in a nest with one of them, for goodness sake! I had to push the darn thing out of the way just to get at an egg. I was afraid I was going to get pecked to death! Just thought I should let you know."

As she drove away, tires crunching on the gravel, Hugh muttered, "Like the wicked witch of the West, or was it the East?" He smiled at that silly woman's comments. Like a bird no bigger than her hand could peck her to death. "I didn't know Eliza was such a pansy," he said loud enough for his wife to hear. "How about you, woman? Did you know Eliza was a pansy?"

CRITTERS

There was no response, which was just fine. He already knew the answer anyway.

After double checking that the barn was ready for what was to come, Hugh led Betty back out of the barn and headed for the coop to check on the "killer bird." By then, the chickens were heading out of the building, anticipating the food that would soon be scattered all around.

Once in the coop, Betty made no move to look in the box for her Boy. When Hugh glanced in himself, he found the box empty. He scanned the small building until he found the bird sitting on a two-by-four overhead.

Hugh felt an odd sense of relief but didn't point the bird out to her. Instead, he put a large bit in the drill and began boring a couple holes the size of a half dollar through the front of building. When that was finished, he stood back a couple feet to make sure the holes were big enough for a bird to get through. Then he went outside and gathered up a few sticks and brought them inside. He pulled out his pocketknife and sat down on the shelf next to Betty to whittle the two short sticks smooth and to just the right length. Picking up the power tool again, he drilled twice more into the wall, but this time tiny, shallow holes. After placing the sticks tightly into the holes, he turned to Betty and asked if she thought her Boy would like them.

Before she could react to the magic word, Hugh heard the roar of a truck engine coming down the driveway and took Betty's arm before she was ready.

"No!" she said adamantly, her face daring defiance.

"Okay, you can stay here, but I'll be right outside." Hugh gave in, hurrying out of the coop.

Chod and Dude Kremer, Fara's younger brothers, were climbing out of a dusty GMC truck. Hugh had always assumed that Chod and Dude were nicknames but had never known them by anything other. There had been a third boy in their family, named Chicory, like the coffee. Everyone called him Chick for short. He died in a farm accident when he was seven.

"Morning boys," Hugh said to the sixty-something gentle giants who came around the front of the truck to greet him with warm smiles and strong handshakes.

These men had been young boys when their parents were killed in a car accident. Fara, who was in tenth grade at the time, dropped out of school to raise them and take over the duties of the farm. Not only did she raise her brothers, but she turned them into fine men along the way.

Together, the three of them built one of the largest cattle businesses in the state of Iowa, remaining honest and humble throughout, which Hugh believed to be remarkable. He admired them to no end.

Hugh could hear the young animals kicking the inside of the truck bed in protest. Eager for a first look, he walked around to the back of the truck to peek through the wooden side rails, just to make sure they hadn't brought him bulls by mistake.

Grinning, he said, "I think we'll put 'em in the yard for a while, let 'em calm down some. I don't want them kicking down the stalls I just rebuilt."

"Good idea, Hugh," Chod said, smiling, then added, "Fara's right behind us with the hay."

"Well then, I'd better get busy and put some coffee on. I know how Fara's gotta have her caffeine." He waited politely for them to finish chuckling before he said, "Just give me a couple of minutes guys."

The two men watched as Hugh disappeared into the chicken coop, reappearing seconds later with Betty in tow.

"Hi there, Betty Lou," Dude said as he slowly walked over and placed a large hand on her shoulder. Betty Lou was one of those childhood nicknames that stuck to her like glue, connecting her forever with the people of her past.

Betty stood at attention as the wheels in her head struggled to turn. Her eyes searched Dude's face for something familiar, then she turned and did the same with Chod.

Out of respect, no one said a word while the woman struggled. They knew she had trouble. After a few minutes of this, Betty tugged on Hugh's arm, letting him know that she was ready to move on.

"Take your time, Hugh," Dude hollered as the couple walked towards the house. "We'll unload those crazy critters." A deep, hearty laugh followed, fading away as he and Betty entered the kitchen.

Hugh helped Betty into a chair at the table while he brewed a pot of coffee for Fara. The rich aroma filled the otherwise stale air in the house. He stood at the window and watched the boys back the truck up to the gate. He wanted to be out there with them something terrible. Then he watched as another truck stacked with hay bales drove in and parked in front of the barn. The driver's door opened and out from behind the wheel came Fara, her pipe hanging out one side of her mouth. He watched her jump down from the truck like she was a kid and then almost lose her balance when her feet hit the ground. "Stubborn old coot," he said out loud.

FARA, THE RIGHT STUFF

He was so excited that he paced the floor, waiting for the coffee to finish brewing. Fara walked in through the kitchen door like she owned the place. The men's coveralls she wore were rolled up at the ankles, exposing her small work boots. On top of a thick head of gray hair was her signature red hat. Rarely were her goofy outfits void of that small, floppy red hat.

You would never have guessed by looking at her that this solid little woman was nearing eighty. Her crooked fingers could still split an apple in half—something she did often to entertain the young men at the church BBQ's. She'd bet five dollars per apple, gloating with a sly glance in their direction the following Sunday as she dropped the money into the donation plate.

She never married, but everyone from around these parts knew Fara'd been in love. They knew she loved a man that she could never have, one she'd met doing business at the cattle auctions. He was married and a professional in both business and empty promises. Why she hung in there with him for all those years, only she could say. Their affair lasted thirty years before he got

109

killed in a car accident, along with his wife and two teenage daughters. A train hit their car one spring morning, splitting it in half and leaving debris and four lifeless bodies along the iron tracks and sprouting fields.

That was the only time in all the years that Hugh had known Fara for her to ask for anything. She sought him and Betty out, needing to be away from town and all the eyes that bored into her broken soul. It was painful to watch a strong person like Fara fall apart; it made her friends feel inadequate and helpless. All she wanted was a safe place to be with her anger and her grief, so Hugh and Betty walked her out into the blooming prairie, and stood quietly at her side for hours, watching as she vacillated between heart wrenching grief and fits of anger. They cringed every time she screamed *fuck*—the mother of all curse words—over the vast landscape. She didn't stop until her voice was hoarse and her body limp with exhaustion.

Then, without saying a word, Fara stuck her pipe in her mouth, took hold of each of their hands and squeezed. Not letting go, she led them back to her truck, where she climbed in and drove away.

Everyone had known about the affair, but no one talked about it, at least not that Hugh had ever heard. Neither did he nor Betty ever ask about it, either before or after the accident. They figured it was none of their business.

Hugh remembered feeling privileged that she'd come to them with her crazy rampage. He was honored that she trusted them and chose their fields to scream at like a drunken sailor.

Looking at her now, Hugh smiled at the memory. "You tough old bird, you," he said to the woman seated next to his wife.

"Takes one to know one, buddy," she said as Hugh set the steaming cup down in front of her.

"How you doing, girl?" Fara asked, reaching over and touching Betty's frail, motionless hand where it was lying on the table. Then, pointing out the window, she added, "You see them calves out there, honey? They're wild ones. I couldn't wait to get 'em off my hands, that's for damn sure." Fara smiled at Hugh and added a wink when he joined them at the table.

Betty was silent, her gaze distracted by the window, but she responded with a smile each time Fara spoke.

Though one couldn't tell by looking at her, Fara was worth millions of dollars, as were her brothers. Years of hard work and good decisions paid off for these small-town kids who'd become wealthy on their own sweat and tears.

When her lover died, she was as shocked as everyone else to find out that he had willed his Cement Company to her. It was a successful business that generated big money, which she used to keep hundreds of people in this small town employed, as well as creating more jobs by building Silver Woods—the assisted living complex in Ottumwa. She planned to donate it as a not-for-profit once it was fully on its feet and running.

She set up a trust for the public schools in Ottumwa, so they would always be able to purchase new buses and improvements when needed. She did the same with the food shelf, keeping it always in food, including delivering fresh meat from her ranch once every month. She even started the very first Meals on Wheels program in Wapello County. There was no question that her wealth gave her loss some purpose.

She's known by the locals—kids and grownups alike—as "Aunt Fara," which she considers the highest honor of her life. Although it is true that she drinks and swears like a sailor on leave, never do you hear an ill word spoken about the woman in the red hat.

After a couple cups of coffee and some updating, Fara rose. "Come on old girl, let's go see what the guys are up to out there." She helped Betty stand up, laced fingers with her, and walked her out of the house.

Hugh remained at the table for a minute, reflecting on their long friendship with Fara and her brothers. Before joining the others, he took the time to apologize to the not-so-unfair God above for his fluctuating faith.

Once outside, he found everyone standing around the fence watching the two little calves work the devil out of themselves by running around the yard. Eileen and Jacob were pulling in just in time to witness the boisterous sight.

The car had barely come to a complete stop when Jacob opened the door and came running up to the fence. "Two of them! Oh, Grandpa, two of them! They're perfect, thank you! Thank you, thank you!" he said, squeezing Hugh tightly.

Thoroughly enjoying the happiness pouring out of his grandson, and the warmth of his short arms around his waist, he reluctantly took hold of the scrawny arms, pulling him just far enough away that he could look down at the excited boy. "Jacob, these calves are a gift from Aunt Fara, so it's her you need to thank."

Jacob immediately released his grip on his Grandpa and ran over to the fence where Fara leaned, hugging her tight. "Thank you, Aunt Fara," he said.

After a couple minutes, she peeled him off her and looked into his teary eyes. "Okay, boy, now this is some serious business you've got going on here. Those four-legged creatures are not toys, ya hear? You got to take care, real good care, of them. You understand?"

"I will Aunt Fara, I promise. I love them so much already!" he said, backing away from her with his head towards the ground. He pretended to walk right past

Chod and Dude, then at the last second, surprised them both with a quick squeeze each.

Eager to get in the yard with his new little buddies, Jacob started walking back to the gate, passing his Grandma on the way. She stood alone and silent near a fence post, watching the calves. All eyes were on him when he did a 180-degree turn and took a hold of her by the waist. He said nothing, just hung onto her. The group watched Betty's limp arms come alive, leaving her side and circling Jacob's little shoulders and neck. Then she rested her head on top of his for the longest time.

It was a tender moment, which brought tears to the eyes of all who witnessed the tender miracle. After a few minutes, Fara broke the silence. "I'm not getting any younger. So, let's get our asses in gear and get that hay unloaded before winter shows up!"

Trading the tears for laughter, they all got busy. It was late afternoon by the time the Kremers said their goodbyes, leaving only a few good hours of daylight to unload the car and trailer stuffed with Eileen and Jacob's things.

Hugh sat Betty in a weathered wicker chair outside the kitchen door, near one of many unattended flower beds, she was safe there and could watch the comings and goings. She made eye contact each time they passed by and greeted them with a "hello" as if every time were the first. The three of them returned her greetings, never tiring of the number of times they said it. They were all having fun.

When the car and trailer were completely empty, Eileen announced that it was time for supper. Hugh and Jacob high-fived each other in triumph for the good day's work and in anticipation of filling their bellies with something yummy.

Having assumed the day would be a long one, Eileen had stopped at the local Kentucky Fried Chicken before heading out to the farm. She had purchased a huge bucket of crispy chicken, a tub of coleslaw, and plenty of biscuits with honey—all of which was consumed at warp speed.

Not surprisingly, the only one with any energy left was Jacob. "Can I put the calves in the barn now, mom?" he asked, pushing his chair away from the table.

Eileen looked to Hugh for input. He nodded 'yes' but added, "I'll be out in a minute to help you bud. Locking that gate is tricky; I want to make sure you see how I do it. We don't want your girls to get loose now do we?"

"No, we sure don't, Grandpa. Okay, I'll just fart around outside and wait for you," he said.

"Sounds good," Hugh said, chuckling at Jacob's choice of words as he watched him skip through the kitchen and disappear out the door.

Eileen offered to change Betty's clothes and get her ready for bed so Hugh could get outside before it got to dark.

"There'll be plenty of time for that, honey. Thanks for the offer, but I'll take care of it," he said, offering her a smile filled with warmth and gratitude.

Once Hugh had changed Betty into her night clothes, he sat her down in the familiar worn leather chair. From there she could watch what was left of the sun slip behind the large oak or watch Eileen as she cleaned up in the kitchen.

He knew Eileen was capable of taking care of Betty, and anything else for that matter, yet he thought it a good idea that she observed their routine before she dived into the caretaking duties.

Routines were necessary. He'd come to understand how necessary they were to a person who was lost most of their waking hours. Betty wasn't the only one who needed routine, it was the only medicine Hugh required.

The old barn was huge and mostly empty. It was cool and damp and smelled of the hundred or so years it had existed. There were good intentions for the lumber that was stacked up here and there. A pot belly stove stood awkwardly off to one side, away from the hay lofts—cold and dusty from years of non-use. The double doors were solid like the many who had passed its threshold. Inside the doors to the left were the stalls Hugh had built to house the new calves.

Hugh and Jacob successfully secured the calves in their new stalls, then dumped grain in their boxes and hauled a couple of buckets of water from the hand pump located in a corner of the barn. When they were finishing up, Hugh turned to Jacob and asked, "Have you thought about what you are going to name them, son?"

Immediately, Jacob pointed to the larger one with spots. It was obvious he had been thinking about it. "That one is Daisy, and I think I'll call the black one Charlotte," he answered.

"How would you feel about calling the black one Bob?" Hugh suggested.

Laughing, Jacob said, "Bob's a boy's name, Grandpa—duh."

Hugh returned the sassy interjection with a large smile. "Once upon a time, your dad had a bull named Bob, did you know that?"

Jacob raised his brows and shook his head.

"Your dad and Grandma loved him more than any of the other critters on the farm, and that's saying a lot because they loved all the critters. I was thinking about how your Grandma might just like to have another Bob around this place. But it's up to you. Whatever you name them is okay with me. Just think about it."

GRANDMA

Jacob turned an empty bucket upside down and sat. He leaned his forehead against the stall so he could watch the calves through the slits in the wood. "What's wrong with Grandma anyway?" he asked unexpectedly.

Hugh sucked in a big breath and let it out slowly. "Well son, your Grandma has a disease called dementia. It's a disease that slowly takes away your memories. You know that game you play on your thingamajig—Pac Man?"

Jacob nodded.

Hugh scratched his head, trying to put his thoughts in order. "Well, imagine those little guys are the disease, cruising around in your brain, eating up everything you know and remember. It's kind of like that. Does that make any sense?"

Jacob gasped, but nodded again. "That's awful," he said, looking up at his Grandpa.

"Yes, it is son, it's worse than awful. Most days she doesn't even talk, or seem to know who I am. And she's only going to get worse, so don't be surprised when your Grandma does or says things that seem a little weird."

"Like what?" Jacob asked.

"Well, let's see. For example, um, she might think you're your dad at times, or even that you're someone else entirely. She's been going back and forth lately, between being a little girl to being a young mother. What is left of her memory seems to be of the past, long ago stuff. Very little of her memory is of anything or anyone recent. More than likely, honey, she doesn't even know that you exist. I don't think she can remember that your dad grew up and became a man, or that he died, which is a blessing in a way. It's hard to explain, but no matter what your Grandma says or does, it's really important that you not be afraid of her, you hear me?"

Hugh stroked Jacob's face. "I could go on, son, but I think you get the point. Her train runs off its tracks and has a hard time getting back on." To lighten the mood, he added, "Just the other day, I heard her answer the phone, and when I walked into the room, she was holding that statue of Roy Rogers to her ear and talking into it!" Hugh's lips formed a crooked smile remembering the sight.

Jacob smiled too. "I'm not afraid of Grandma," he said. "I think she's funny, and besides—I love her."

"You sweet thing, she loves you too. Just remember that trapped inside of her is the same wonderful person we've always known."

Hugh's head turned towards the hay loft and his eyes searched beyond the rafters for the invisible presence of God. "Thank you," he whispered.

When his eyes returned to Jacob, he found empathy and understanding reflected on his young face. Hugh couldn't help but grab hold of the boy and give him a kiss on the head. He choked back tears, and as he released him, said, "Okay, that's enough of that. Now, before we call it quits for the night, there's someone I want you to meet."

On their way out of the barn, Jacob said, "Bob's a good name for the black one, Grandpa."

With a smile pasted on the old man's face, he and his grandson made their way to the chicken coop. The night was blissfully quiet, and the oncoming winter rode on the breeze. Hugh was ready for winter now; in fact, he was ready for anything that came his way.

"Who the heck am I going to meet in the chicken coop, Grandpa?" Jacob asked as they entered the small building.

"You'll see in a minute, boy." Hugh chuckled. *Boy meets boy*, he thought to himself.

It was nearly too dark inside the coop to see anything, so Hugh pulled on the string that hung from the bulb on the wall, illuminating the space in a yellowish glow.

He peeked into Boy's box and started laughing when he saw Mrs. Nickels asleep in it. She lazily opened one eye and looked up at him.

"What the devil are you doing in here?" he asked the groggy cat.

Curious, Jacob climbed up on the shelf and looked inside the box. "I can't believe the chickens let her sleep in here, Grandpa."

"Me either," Hugh murmured, busily searching the rest of the boxes until he found what he was looking for on the top shelf, next to a nesting chicken.

"Looky here, Jacob. This is who I wanted you to meet. Let me introduce you to Boy."

Hugh stepped away so Jacob could get a good look. "That looks like the same bird Mrs. Nickels had in her mouth the other day," Jacob said, looking at his grandfather with a questioning expression and an exaggerated twist of his lips.

"That's the one. Your Grandma and I found him a couple weeks ago out in the yard. He hit the window and . . . long story short: your Grandma took a liking to it, so I kept it for her. She calls him Boy." Hugh raised his shoulders and put his palms up to convey it didn't make sense to him either. "The little guy seems to like it in here, though."

"That's crazy," Jacob said, still watching the bird that appeared to be looking back at him.

"Which part, son? It's all crazy if you ask me. What I can't believe is that Mrs. Nickels hasn't made a meal out of the little guy yet, and I sure hope she doesn't. I'm getting kind of used to having him around. So, Boy here is now your responsibility too, and since the bugs will be gone soon, you'll need to keep some birdseed in here for him eat."

"Okay!" Before Jacob climbed down from the shelf to join his Grandpa, he reached over and patted Mrs. Nickels on the head. "Now you leave Boy alone, ya hear?" he ordered the cat.

Grandfather and grandson walked out of the coop and into the house, like it all was just as normal as apple pie on Sunday.

It was quiet and cozy when they entered the house. The aroma of Kentucky Fried Chicken still hung in the air, the only lights that were on came from the one over the kitchen sink and the one by the empty chair, where Betty no longer rested.

Hugh was just about to tell Jacob to get ready for bed when Eileen came down from the second-floor bedroom with an armload of boxes. "I thought you guys got lost out there," she said, smiling. "What were you up to for so long?"

"Just getting the critters settled in for the night, is all," Jacob said, just a bit defensively.

"Oh," his mom responded, giving them both a quizzical look.

"I put Betty to bed a while ago but made sure she was asleep before I went upstairs to unpack. Almost got it done too, so tomorrow I'll start on Jacob's room."

"That's great," Hugh said as his stomach did a flip. He worried that Eileen might not have kept an eye on Betty while so engaged in unpacking. That was why he wasn't going to turn over his duties entirely. He couldn't risk losing his wife ever again. But he knew Eileen meant well, she always meant well.

He hurried to the bedroom, hoping his fear wasn't too obvious, but when he peeked inside the dark room, he saw the lump on the bed and heard a soft snore. His old heart calmed as he registered that all was well.

"Thank you," he said, walking back towards the kitchen. "I'm sorry we weren't around to help you unpack. Right Jacob?" He nudged the boy with his elbow.

"Yeah, me too, mom. Dang it," Jacob said with a grin.

"Okay, time for bed, young man. We can start all over again tomorrow. Now git," Eileen ordered, pushing Jacob gently toward his new room.

"Night mom, night Grandpa, and thanks for everything!" Jacob said with a wink before disappearing into his room.

"What was that all about?" Eileen asked, having noticed the conspiratorial wink.

"You got me," Hugh answered, shrugging. "All I know is that it's time I hit the hay too. See you in the morning, honey." Before he reached his bedroom, he turned and looked at his daughter-in-law. "And thank you again for everything!"

The next morning, Hugh panicked when he looked over and found the space next to him empty. The lump in the bed was gone, and fear seized him once again. He tore his robe off the chair as he ran out of the room, calling, "Wife?" He ran into the living room and called again. "*Wife*?" He could hear that his voice was becoming frantic. Before he got to the kitchen, he was stopped dead in his tracks by the singing that floated down the stairs. It was coming from the bedroom that was now Eileen's, but it wasn't Eileen's voice he heard. It was Betty's.

He took the stairs two at a time, reaching the doorway to the bedroom. He froze in place when he saw her sitting on the bed, cradling a doll in her arms, and singing the song she'd been humming for weeks.

"*You are my sunshine, my only sunshine, you make me happy when skies are gray*," she sang. Then she reverted to humming a few verses, until she got to, "*Please don't take my sunshine away,*" which she belted out, more like a desperate plea than a song.

Betty held the doll near her face until she finally looked over to Hugh, then held it out to him. "See?" she asked, but after a few seconds she tucked it back up against her chest and continued rocking back and forth. "Boy," she said, smiling down at the worn cloth doll.

Hugh was so relieved that she wasn't wandering around outside that he didn't know whether to laugh or to cry, but he definitely felt like he could do either.

BABY BOY

When Hugh sat on the edge of the bed next to her, Betty immediately reached over and took one of his hands, placing it on the doll. "Boy," she said again, making a point or an introduction, he wasn't sure which. Then she went back to humming.

He nudged in a little closer, placing his free arm around her thin shoulders. As their bodies touched, he could feel her warmth, and before he knew it, tears filled his eyes, spilling over and running down his cheeks. "Yes, Wife. Boy."

At that moment, all he wanted to do was assure the woman sitting next to him that he would never take her sunshine away, ever. But there was no point in telling her that, and he knew it.

Eileen came rushing up the stairs with Jacob trailing her, the pair of them sounding like a herd of elephants. The noise gave Hugh enough leeway to wipe the tears from his face before his daughter-in-law was there, hesitating in the doorway. She evaluated the scene before taking a few short steps into the room, leaving a sleepy Jacob behind her. Then, she bent down and dug into one of her boxes, her hand coming out with a little plastic baby bottle. She looked at Hugh with compassion before handing the bottle to Betty, who eagerly accepted it and began feeding the doll.

"I'll go make some breakfast. You guys come on down when you're ready, okay?" Eileen said, taking Jacob by the arm on her way out.

Hugh stared at the empty doorway, listening to the sound of their bare feet on the wooden stairs. It had been a long time since he heard that sound—since the house was alive—and he was grateful for the noise. He also felt appreciation for how Eileen jumped right in and went along with Betty, no matter what.

He looked over at his woman—his partner and friend of a lifetime, the mother of their only child—and saw something in her face that he hadn't seen in an exceptionally long time: peace.

Only when his arm started to grow numb did he lower it to her waist and usher Betty and "child" off the bed towards the stairs.

Rays from the early morning sun darted in and out of the dirty bedroom window as they passed. By the time they crested the top step, the wonderful smell of sausage and cakes found them. They entered the kitchen just as Eileen had finished filling their plates. Hugh helped his wife into a chair at the table, and when Eileen came near, he whispered, "Thank you."

"No need for that, Hugh," she said, looking into his tear-filled eyes. "I get it, I really do, and it's going to be all right. Trust me."

"I do trust you, honey, and I'm so damned glad you're here I can hardly stand it," he said, as Jacob walked into the room wearing an old pair of Charly's pants. They were so big on him it was hard not to laugh—and laugh they did. It's true that timing is everything.

As Eileen set the plates on the table, Hugh went to the hall closet and pulled out a pair of suspenders, attaching them to his grandson's trousers. "There boy, now you look like a real farmer," he said.

"Awesome," Jacob said, admiring himself in the full-length mirror attached to the closet door.

"Now, let's join Grandma and her Boy at the table."

Hearing that, Betty looked up and smiled. It was going to be a great day. Hugh could feel it.

BOY

I had no complaints, other than the furry one taking over my nest. It was turning out to be not such a bad place to spend the winter. It sure beat the cramped hole of a tree, or the usual tangle of musty grass.

In fact, the other night, when the wind blew in through the cracks, my bed partner even made sure I was safe and warm all night.

I had plenty to eat, a nest to sleep in—even if I do have to share it. Plus, I knew I had friends that would protect me if I needed, making me feel pretty darn good.

I'm even fairly certain that the furry one has joined my team if you can believe that.

Wife hasn't been to see me for a while, but a shorter, little guy has. If I could learn to trust him as well, then maybe I could put my fears to rest for a few more months.

ANOTHER CLOSE CALL

During breakfast, Jacob looked over at his mom, wondering why they hadn't gone to church like they usually did on Sundays. He wanted to ask but was afraid that if he brought it up, she would make them go, and the plans he had for the day would be ruined.

He was eager to get outside and get his chores done so he could spend the rest of the day with his new calves. He hurried through his stack of pancakes, deciding to keep his curiosity about church to himself, when suddenly his Grandma started to cough and choke on a bite of sausage.

Eileen jumped up and ran around the table. "Betty are you all right?" she cried, noticing that the coughs had stopped and she didn't seem to be getting any air. With the heel of her hand, Eileen gave several hard blows to her bony back. When that didn't seem to help, she put two fingers in the old woman's mouth, hoping to grab whatever had blocked her airway.

Betty's confused, terrified eyes bulged from their sockets and Hugh stood up, unsure what to do. "How can I help!?" he cried.

"Try to stay calm, Hugh," Eileen said, cool and firm, as she removed her fingers from Betty's mouth. "I know first aid."

Still seated, Jacob watched in horror as his grandmother's face turned a faint shade of purple. His mother moved behind Betty's chair to lift her from it. She then jammed her fist into his grandmother's abdomen, which scared him even more.

After a few stomach thrusts on Betty's little abdomen, a chunk of Jimmy Dean sausage flew out, landing on the linoleum floor with a thud. Mrs. Nickels appeared out of nowhere and took care of the mess in a hurry.

Within seconds of having her life saved by the daughter-in-law she no longer recognized, Betty was back in her chair, rocking and humming to her Boy, as if nothing had happened.

Hugh kissed the top of Betty's gray head in relief. He felt angry at being so helpless, and not knowing what to do.

Eileen saw the pain written on his face. "Hugh, help me out with the dishes, would you?" she asked. She put the dirty dishes in the sink, careful not to look at him when he moved in next to her.

"Thank God you knew what to do," he said. "I can't help thinking about what would have happened if you hadn't been here."

Searching for the right words to calm and reassure him, she said, "You can't know how to do everything. I'm trained in first aid and CPR, that's part of why I'm here—to help you. Come on, we're a team now, remember?" She turned away from the window to face him, his tall lanky frame towering next to her. "When I was in college, one of the things I had to study was different types of diseases and how they attack, not only animals, but people too. Dementia and Alzheimer's are two of the crippling brain diseases I focused on. Charly was interested in all of it too. He was in most of my classes, that's actually when we started to date."

She smiled after sharing that with him, and so did Hugh, but his fear-filled expression didn't change. "I don't claim to be an expert," Eileen continued. "But I do remember a few things that I'd like to tell you about. Okay with you?"

He nodded.

"As you might know, some people with dementia wander. It's a trait of the disease that I didn't realize Betty had until recently. So, I promise you from here on out, I'll be much more aware of where Betty is when I'm alone with her."

Fearing Eileen was feeling guilty, Hugh started to say something, but Eileen plunged ahead before he could get a word in. "I also know that choking is something that happens in the later stages of this disease. It's a sign she no longer remembers to chew her food."

Hugh backed up a few feet, but never took his eyes off her.

"In nursing homes, when a patient gets to this point, they puree their food, so maybe that's something we should do. I also know that some women, the ones who were mothers, go through a period where they search for their children. As they regress in age, so do their memories of people in their lives, particularly of their children. So, they search. When I saw Betty with my old doll, I knew right away what it represented to her. That's why I gave her the baby bottle." Eileen smiled. Then she went on, cautiously. "A few days ago, when I was cleaning out Charly's room, I found some photos of him. When Betty saw them, I could tell she recognized him. She pointed to him in each photo and called him *Boy*."

Hugh nodded, confirming that what she was telling him was something he was already aware of.

Eileen continued, "When I heard her call that bird the same name, I put two and two together. She's searching for something in her past, a time when she was a mother, when she took care of someone, or something—like her son or the animals on the farm."

He understood what she was saying and didn't disagree. When she finished talking, the two of them just stood at the counter, looking out the window. "Just remember this, Old Man," she said, breaking their silence. "We can handle anything as a team. Anything." Their foreheads came together and touched, sealing the deal.

"Mom?" Jacob said, coming into the kitchen and abruptly ending the private moment. "Didn't you used to sing that same song to me? The one Grandma's humming?"

"I sure did, honey. Do you want me to sing it to you right now?"

"No way, Jose! All I want to do is go outside!" he said, as he headed for the door. "I'm going to feed the chickens, Grandpa, and anything else that's living in there." He gave his grandfather a sly wink. "I'll be in the barn."

"I'll be out in a few minutes," Hugh said, winking back. But the boy was long gone by then.

By the time Jacob got to the coop, the chickens were already outside, pecking at the bare ground. He couldn't wait to see who, or what, was in the coop, and was disappointed when he found it empty. As instructed, he placed birdseed in the windowsill, then searched the small building one more time. Still finding no sign of Boy, he went about the chore of cleaning out the poop, replacing it with sawdust and a little straw. Then he hurriedly scattered the feed for the hungry chickens and took off running towards the barn, tripping on the pant legs made for someone much taller and bigger than he was.

He noticed Mrs. Nickels perched on top of a nearby fence post, watching him, and walked over to her.

"Good morning, Mrs. Nickels," he said, stroking her head and silky body. The cat's tail flipped back and forth in pleasure. "I sure hope you didn't eat that little bird for breakfast or you're going to be in some deep shit."

Inside the house, Hugh sat at the table with a fresh cup of tea, watching Betty happily rock her baby Boy.

Eileen grabbed her cup of coffee off the counter and joined them, saying, "You know, Thanksgiving's right around the corner. How would you feel about inviting a few people out to the farm? Make it a real old-fashioned Thanksgiving?"

It had been a long time since Hugh and Betty celebrated a real Thanksgiving meal, much less entertained dinner guests. The thought of it warmed him.

November did that to people. The skies changed along with the air, and darkness slowly took over the light. Barren fields transformed themselves in stages, ending in a snow-covered landscape—impressions in the powder showing clues as to what creatures lived and traveled there.

Hugh asked, "What do you think, Wife? Want to invite some people out here for Thanksgiving?"

Betty looked at him, her blue eyes flickering with life, but there was no response.

He didn't mind, the flicker was enough for him. Suddenly he became aware of all the things he was thankful for.

His expression answered Eileen's question, but he gave her arm a little squeeze anyway. "Sounds like a wonderful idea, honey. Tell me what you want me to do."

"Just get that barrel stove in the barn working and leave the rest to me. I'm so excited Hugh, it's going to be the best Thanksgiving ever!"

He was elated to see Eileen happy. A gathering of people they loved, and the idea of a true Thanksgiving feast might just be what the doctor ordered.

Hugh led Betty to the chair by the window, as he did every morning for more months than he could count. But this time she refused to sit down. When he tried to encourage her to bend at the waist, she stiffened and straightened her crooked body. This was new. Puzzled, he bent down and looked into her eyes, hoping they would give him a clue as to where she was. When he did, she returned his look, mocking him, then she started to laugh. He couldn't help but laugh himself.

"You think this is funny, do you?" he asked, still trying to bend her stiff frame into the chair.

"Yes," she answered.

Shocked, Hugh let go of her, but then quickly grabbed her and held her against his chest. He justified his quick movements with the knowledge that the moment of familiarity was already evaporating.

Betty's arms were trapped against his belly. As he ate up their closeness, she tried to pull away, so he released his grip and backed up. Betty indicated to the bundle of cloth she cradled in one arm but said nothing. Her eyes and pointing finger said it all: she was worried that they were going to crush the baby. She was still in this world with him — sort of — which amazed him.

"Oh, of course, the boy. I'm sorry," he said, stroking the bundle she held out for him to see. Hugh could hardly contain the tangle of emotions running through him. He glanced over at the table where Eileen sat. She offered no assistance, as it was clear to her that none was needed. Instead, she looked back at him, grinning, both amused and touched.

Hugh turned back to his wife and said, "Let's go see how Daisy and Bob are doing on this fine morning, shall we?" He placed a sweater over her shoulders and led her out of the house.

Still grinning, Eileen got up, poured herself another cup of coffee, and then began making the guest list for their Thanksgiving dinner.

Outside, as the couple strolled through the maze of pecking chickens, Hugh noticed that Betty took no interest in the chicken coop as they passed. They continued down the lane towards the barn, passing Mrs. Nickels. The cat sat motionless on a post, watching the nearby open field, ready to pounce on the slightest movement.

Betty also paid no attention to the cat who hunted like a perched hawk, but Hugh did. He couldn't help himself and greeted their old friend with a "hello." The preoccupied cat ignored them—muscles tense and glittering eyes focused.

They left the daylight and entered the dim and dusty barn, where a sweet little voice was coming from one of the stalls.

"You are my sunshine, my only sunshine."

Hugh stopped and listened to the sweet, melodious voice—and so did Betty.

"You make me happy when skies are gray. You'll never know dear . . ."

Betty broke away from Hugh and walked towards the stall where Jacob was sitting on the ground with his arm around the calf named Daisy. She joined in the singing, not missing a beat.

". . . how much I love you. Please don't take my sunshine away."

Jacob looked up at his grandmother and smiled. She smiled back at him, and right then something came fluttering down from the rafters and landed on Betty's shoulder. It was Boy, the bird.

Hugh stood alone, watching as the crazy miracle unfolded before him, knowing that no matter how hard he tried, he would never be able to describe it to anyone.

One more time, he found himself searching past the rafters for the invisible presence he held so much faith in. He knew right then that the ones he really wanted to share the miracles with had already witnessed, if not handed them to him.

The rest of the day was spent outside, with no more sign of Boy. After they brought the calves out to the yard, he flew away to do whatever it was birds do. Hugh cleaned out the wood stove in the barn, as requested by Eileen, hauling in firewood with his four-wheeler and cart, until there was enough wood to stay the winter.

Betty and baby rode in front of Hugh, sharing the one seat while he worked, and even though there was heat in the autumn sun, the air was still cool. Every once in a while, Hugh reached around to wipe her runny nose with his hanky. He added one of his flannel shirts to her sweater to make sure she stayed warm and toasty. One of his biggest fears was Betty getting sick with fever.

He remembered how afraid he was when the year before she was sick with a cold and high fever. He took her to town to see Doctor Spevak, and before they left his office with instructions, advice, and plenty of antibiotics, he pulled Hugh aside, out of earshot of Betty.

"You know what we call pneumonia in the old and the sick, Hugh? We call it the old man's friend. Do you know what I mean by that?"

He did know. Doc was saying that dying in your sleep from pneumonia isn't the worst thing that can happen to a person who is slowly dying anyway. He was saying that it was a blessing to those who suffer from whatever it is that brutally steals their life away from them.

Hugh hoped instead that God would take her away easily when the time came, but not by a fever which he had the choice to treat or not to treat. At that time, he wasn't certain that Betty was truly suffering with dementia. Failing fast, yes, but not suffering. Hell, *he* was suffering, but no one was talking about him.

It was her fate that was being broached by the doctor—he'd known him since the man was a boy in elementary school and in 4-H. Hell, Betty and Hugh had even attended the doc's high school graduation ceremony.

Hugh trusted this man, cared for him even, but he was not ready or willing to talk about letting his wife die.

"I hear what you're saying, Doc, but she's not ready, and I'm not ready either, okay? I'll call you if she needs any more antibiotics. Thanks," Hugh said as he guided his wife through the office doors.

"Take care Hugh, you too, Betty Lou," the doctor said, watching the two bent frames slowly walk out of the clinic.

Faith and love led him through that next few months, and the fear of being without her dictated his days.

As he reminisced, he enjoyed the warm feeling of her against him—her heart beating on his chest while they rode. She hadn't said another word since joining Jacob in song that morning, and for the first time in a long time, the silence was beautiful.

They hadn't been this kind of close in years. It was the best of the best. As he soaked it up, he promised himself from then on, that if any words came from her mouth—no matter how mixed up—they would be a gift he wouldn't take for granted. Her complete silence was just over the horizon and he knew it.

The old four-wheeler roared down the long driveway towards the mailbox, hitting a deep rut in the road, making both their butts leave the seat for a split second. Hugh didn't notice the doll had fallen from Betty's grasp when they hit the hole. He only realized it when Betty began to stand up, making him stop a little too quickly. They both lost their balance, but just before they tumbled off, he was able to hit the kill switch, bringing the machine to a slow halt a few feet ahead of them.

They landed in the road on their backs behind the four-wheeler, both looking into the cold sky, dazed. With his heart in his throat, Hugh jumped up from the hard ground—not so easy for a person of his age—and hurried over to Betty. She'd landed farther to the right of the vehicle and lay flat on the ground, wiry gray hair spilling away from her face as she smiled up at him.

"Are you all right?" he asked, kneeling next to his wife. He put his hand under her back to help her sit up, but she shook her head in refusal. Then, with one hand, she grabbed his jacket and attempted to pull him down closer to her, while her other hand patted the gravel beside where she lay.

Confused, he did as instructed, and sat down beside her. She continued to smile and pat the ground until he realized that what she wanted was for him to lie down next to her, which he did. Once he was down, he put his left arm under her head as a pillow, and she moved her head onto his chest, nestling into him. "Love you," he heard her say.

He lay on the hard, cold ground, holding his wife's body next to his, and began to laugh. The hearty laughter spread to his wife like a contagion, and they were both chuckling when they heard a truck approaching. It came to a speedy halt on the road behind them, spraying loose gravel as it did.

Hugh heard a door slam shut, the sound of footsteps, then much huffing and puffing before, "Oh my God! Oh my God!"

Standing over them was Leroy Graham, their mailman. His face was as white as the curly hair that stuck out the sides of his red and black checkered hat. "Hugh, what the hell man? Are you two okay? I mean, when I saw your four-wheeler and then you lying here, I about shit my pants. Do you want me to call for help?"

"No, Leroy, we're okay, but if you could go get the baby in the road, and bring it back to us, I sure would appreciate it," Hugh said, pointing.

"A baby? Oh my God, Hugh, what's going on?" Leroy cried, running as fast as he could up the driveway to where the doll lay in the ditch on its side. Relieved, he walked slowly back to the two bodies laughing and cuddling in the road. He shook his head, trying to regain some sanity, as he handed the doll to them.

All humor aside, Hugh was glad to see the color returning to Leroy's face. He felt bad for the man, knowing he was shaken up.

"Are you sure you don't want me to call someone? I mean, it's no problem. At least let me help you guys up," Leroy offered.

The clouds moved over, covering the sun, and a light snow began to fall.

"No, we're good, Leroy. Eileen's at the house. Trust me, we're good right where we are. But if you don't mind, would you do me one last favor and bring us the mail?"

Leroy stood still for a few more seconds. "It's Sunday Hugh, ain't no mail today. I was just on my way over to Evert's to watch a football game, and I just happened to look up your driveway and . . . hell man, you scared me to death."

From the ground, Hugh offered an apology. "I'm sorry, Leroy. I sure didn't mean to. I appreciate you stopping, I really do. Now you go on and watch that football game and tell Evert we said hello."

Turning towards his truck, the slightly less ashen mailman said, "Okay then. I guess I'll be seeing ya."

It was a few more minutes before Hugh heard Leroy shut the truck door and start the engine. He knew they were being watched, so he stifled his laughter until the man was gone.

After another ten minutes or so, their laughing evaporated, and he sensed that she had left that place of togetherness. He stood her up to dust her off and assess any possible damage. Finding none, he loaded them back on the four-wheeler and headed towards home.

Fun, that's what that was, he thought. *Fun, fun, fun*. Hugh chuckled, thinking about how crazy it must have looked with the two of them lying in the road. He chuckled even more when he thought of how mail carriers were like barbers: soon everyone in town who knew them, and even those who didn't, would hear of their little episode. But he didn't care, he was so friggin' happy.

BOY

The first day I could stand without feeling that stabbing pain, I decided to test out my landing skills by flying around the fields, alighting here and there on fence posts and barren branches.

I flew in and out of the naked trees, dodging the harassing black giants who scavenge the fields for bits of corn. They were big, and their red eyes threatened me every time I flew past them.

Personally, I don't like corn. I didn't know how I knew this, but I did. They could have the dry, old corn for all I care. What I did know is that the danger I felt around them was familiar. I knew in my gut that they were my enemies and meant harm, just as I knew I didn't like corn. It's a feeling I thought I'd better pay attention to.

Satisfied, but feeling danger from the black giants, I flew back to the safety of my new winter home. On my way, I saw the furry one sleeping in the sun near the fence line. I thought, Why not? *So, I joined her.*

She didn't protest in the least when I landed on her back and nestled into her soft fur. We both snoozed in the sun until a loud growling in my belly woke me up. She must have been hungry too, because when I took off towards my house, she followed.

We made it home just as the sky started to throw small white balls to the ground. My other bird friends rushed inside as fast as they could, and the furry one was right behind them.

I have to admit that I'm thankful for not having to live in the fields, or the trees, just yet. I'm grateful to the Old Man and Wife for having saved me.

THAT'S IOWA FOR YA

The temperature began to drop as the snow fell upon the farm. This snow wouldn't last. It never did this time of year in Iowa. As they entered the kitchen, Hugh thought back to when they were kids and how excited they were at the first snow. He remembered how, by the time they gathered up their warm clothes, found their sleds and headed outside, the snow had already begun to melt.

He chuckled, "That's Iowa for ya."

The smell of homemade chili and cornbread filled the house, and the falling snow made everything inside that much warmer and cozier.

Jacob sat at the table, peeling off his work clothes, while Eileen tugged at one end of his leg, grunting as she tried to remove one muddy boot clinging to his sweaty foot. In between her groans, she delivered a scolding for not taking his boots off at the door.

Hugh winked as he passed his grandson on his way to aid his wife, removing the flannel shirt and sweater from her shoulders. She didn't help much as he maneuvered around the soiled baby doll and pried the clothing away from her stiff arms. Before heading to the kitchen to make them something warm to drink, he wiped his wife's runny nose and patted Eileen on the shoulder.

"I was just thinking of sending out a search party to look for you two. Where the heck were you all this time, Hugh?" Eileen asked.

Hugh couldn't help but grin. "I guess I can't keep track of what day it is anymore. I thought it was a mail day, so we went to pick it up. When I figured out it was Sunday and there was no mail, we farted around at the end of the driveway until it started to snow. It took a little longer than I'd expected." He wanted to add that she was sure to be hearing about it soon enough, but he didn't.

Hugh casually changed the subject by asking Jacob about his day with the calves. They talked back and forth from the dining room to the kitchen, until Jacob was finally free of his boots and standing right next to his Grandpa, looking up at him.

"They're so great Grandpa and really smart! I fed them and started to lead them back to the barn, when they just went right past me, going right into their stalls, like they knew whose was whose. It was awesome."

"That's great son but do me a favor. Don't trust them quite yet—them calves can be sneaky, believe it or not. They're not as smart as you give them credit for. They just learn early on what's called 'repetition.' It's like follow-the-leader. They're creatures of habit, which means that the more they do something, the more it becomes natural for them. Get it?"

"I hear what you're saying Grandpa, but my girls are different!" Jacob said defensively.

On his way back to the table, Hugh put an end to the conversation with his grandson by adding, "Well, who knows, Jacob? Maybe Aunt Fara gave you special ones."

Satisfied, Jacob smiled and nodded in agreement, then headed to his room to change clothes. Before he was out of earshot, Eileen reminded him that he had to take a shower, because the following day was a school day. She wasn't positive, but she thought she heard him say "damn it" as he closed his bedroom door.

Night came fast, and the snow came hard. Everyone devoured the chili and cornbread. Eileen and Jacob headed to their rooms for the night while Hugh sat awhile longer at the table, looking at the woman next to him. Even with her vacant eyes and chili all over her chin, he thought her beautiful. Reaching over, he dabbed at her face with a napkin from the pile wedged inside the blue plastic holder. Charly had made it in Boy Scouts when he was seven out of a plastic detergent jug bought from the Fuller Brush Man. This door-to-door salesman was a common visitor back in the days of past, someone you could count on stopping in once a week, kind of like the Jehovah's Witnesses, but different.

Charly had drawn around his little hands and fingers with a marker on the plastic jug, and with the help of his dad, cut it to make a napkin holder.

Hugh remembered that project and the day they made it and was grateful for the memory. He wondered whether Betty could remember what it was. She was staring at it, but did she know it had been a gift from her son for Mother's Day? He doubted it. Now, it was just something to focus on, to get lost in. And although he felt it was unfair, he was beginning to accept, rather than feel sad.

Over the past few weeks, something in him had shifted. It was an awakening—clarity, one might say—that replaced the sadness and self-pity that had been smothering him. Hugh was no longer going to waste what precious time he had left on this earth being sad or feeling sorry for himself.

Calling it a night, he helped Betty and her doll up from the chair and led them into the bedroom. Across the hall was Jacob's room. His door was open and so were his eyes and ears. Before his Grandpa shut his door, Jacob overheard him tell his Grandma, "Thanks for a great day, Wife."

The next day, Eileen took Jacob to school and let Hugh know that she planned on visiting her parents in their new digs before she returned to the farm.

Hugh's routine with Betty would resume for the time being. He watched the snow drip off the roof and decided to keep Betty inside for a while, at least until things dried out some. The dampness was hard on old bones, and after their excursion the day before, he knew she must be a little sore. He certainly was.

Jacob got up early to feed the chickens and let his buddies out to roam the fenced yard before he headed off to school. When Eileen returned, Hugh would double-check on the critters, just to give him something to do. In the meantime, he sat at the table and watched Betty's chest rise and fall as she slept peacefully in her chair.

Sipping the last bit of tea in his cup, he noticed a pad of paper on the other side of the table. It was the Thanksgiving list.

"Wow," he said, as he looked through the names. There were at least three dozen people written down in his daughter-in-law's neat cursive. Eileen had even included the round bossy one—Eliza. Naturally, next to her name was her husband Charles's, a good man, and a hard-working son of a gun.

Hugh heard that Charles was now delivering pizzas on the weekends for Bambinos, an Italian restaurant in Ottumwa. What he didn't know, not that it was any of his business, was whether Charles did it because he needed the extra money, or because he needed to get out the house. He thought the latter was probably more like it.

He reviewed the list a little longer, realizing how all the names fit into the puzzle he called his life, and he was truly thankful for each and every one of them—even "bossy pants."

Glancing one more time at the list before setting it back on the table, a proverbial light bulb went off, and he immediately knew what his afternoon project would be. With all these people coming, they were going to need tables and benches, so he ripped off a blank sheet of paper from the pad and began sketching. Once the critters were checked on, he would dig into that pile of lumber stacked up in the barn, and maybe even put a fire in the old wood stove so Betty could sit in there while he worked.

Perfect, he thought, just perfect.

BOYS WILL BE BOYS

When Jacob got off the school bus that afternoon, he was mad, storming all the way up the driveway and into the house. He walked through the kitchen door, slamming it behind him and stomping to his room without taking off his coat or boots.

"Hey. Hey, hey, young man," Eileen barked, as she followed him to his room. "Just what the heck has gotten into you?"

Jacob plopped down on the bed and she sat next to him, prepared to give him a lecture. But before she could, he blurted out, "I got into a fight today. I didn't want to, mom, but he stole my damn gloves, and on top of that, Ms. Ashley made ME sit in her office, ME!"

Eileen's face was stricken, both by his news and his favorite swear word, but before she could say anything about either, he went on, "When I went to my locker to get dressed for the bus, my gloves were mysteriously gone! I know it was him because at recess he told me that he didn't have any gloves. I remember that very well, because he was teaching me some new words right before the bell rang. I was so mad. I punched him right in the face!"

"Who is 'him,' honey? Who did you punch in the face?" she asked with urgency.

Jacob looked at his mom and made a snotty face. "Dan. Dan-The-Man, a thief and a big ole bully. Oh, and a liar too. That's what he is."

This was the first time Eileen had heard of her son having conflict with anyone. With her guts in a knot, she tried to think of what to say to calm him down so they could talk about it.

"Nothin' worse than a liar and a thief. That's what you and Grandpa always say, right mom?" Jacob asked defensively.

"Well, yes, that's what we always say, Jacob, but we also say that you shouldn't hit anyone. Remember that part?" his mother countered.

"That's not what Grandpa says. He says that you don't hit anyone 'for no good reason,' and I had a good reason!" he protested, his face getting redder and tears rolling down his cheeks.

"For future reference honey, the only time you have my permission to hit someone is if they are hurting you, and there's no other choice. Got it? And as far as this Dan-The-Man stealing your gloves, I'll handle that. I'll talk to Ms. Ashley tomorrow and get this straightened out."

Mary Ashley was Jacob's fifth grade teacher, and Eileen felt certain she would straighten all of this out.

What bothered her more than her son being in trouble at school was the look on his face. It pained her that she couldn't shield him from the ugly stuff life throws at a child.

She reached for her son's fisted hand, hoping that this turmoil would be the last. But in her heart, she knew it wouldn't be. Unfortunately, it was just the beginning of growing up.

"Hey, why don't you head outside and check on your girls? Grandpa's already out there somewhere. Maybe you can talk to him about this, but only if you want to, okay bud?" Hugging him, and feeling his arms return the hug, lightened the sick feeling in her stomach.

He was almost to the door when Eileen said, "Hey, you didn't tell me what words you learned today."

He turned and answered. "Farming words mom, like 'corn hole' and 'dick weed.' Dan said that dick weed is something that grows all over down south. I'm not sure what corn hole means, but I'll ask Grandpa. He'll know, being a farmer an' all." Then just like that, he was gone.

"Lord!" Eileen exclaimed, when a sound like a giggle came from behind her. She quickly turned around and walked over to the little body lying in the big chair. Betty was still asleep, her eyes closed. Eileen wondered, as she looked down at her, if Betty could dream. And if she could, would her dreams be as mixed up as her waking world? She pondered the question as she pulled up the afghan at the old woman's feet, tucking it tightly against her shoulders and neck. With closed eyes, Betty grinned.

Eileen gently touched one side of Betty's face and whispered, "Sleep well, you little eavesdropper," before walking into the kitchen to make supper.

By the time Jacob got to the barn, his school turmoil was no longer his major concern. He entered at a trot, shutting the large doors behind him.

"Hey Grandpa," he said, walking over to where Hugh was busy measuring boards on a couple sawhorses.

"Hey buddy," his Grandpa answered, not looking up. "Bob and Daisy are out in the east yard where they can stay until we're done here. Come hold this board for me while I cut it. This is the last one," he said, wiping the sweat from his brow and glancing down at his grandson. "You're just in time to help me screw all of this together." He pointed to the large pile of lumber stacked up near the old wood stove that was putting off some serious heat.

"Whoa, is it hot in here or what?" Jacob said, peeling his coat off and flinging it over the side of one of the stalls. "What the heck are you making?"

"What we're making, son, are the tables and benches for our Thanksgiving dinner. Looks like your mom is inviting the whole county out here, and there sure isn't enough room in the house for all of us. We're going to have a feast out here in the barn. What do ya think of them apples?"

"Sounds good to me," Jacob said. Overhead, he suddenly noticed the sign his Grandpa made for him, fixed to one of the beams. "Jacob's Farm" was painted in big, black letters, and seventy-odd years' worth of arrowheads were strategically circling the words. It was beautiful.

"That is so cool, Grandpa. Wow, you made that for me? Thanks a lot. That just turned my shitty day into an awesome one!" he said, staring up at the hand-crafted sign, which hung next to his father's faded one.

"Well, I'm glad you like it son, but you got to knock off that language of yours. You're too damn young to be cussing like that, especially around an adult. It's disrespectful." Hugh walked the few feet to his grandson and put his arms around him. "Hear me, boy? Enough of that, okay?"

"Whatever you say, Grandpa. And thanks a ton, I love it."

The two of them spent the rest of the afternoon and early evening screwing together the tables and benches Hugh cut out of scrap lumber. When the last bench was assembled, Hugh set it underneath a table with the others. Then, they stood back and admired their work.

"Perfect," Hugh said.

"Yep, perfect," Jacob echoed.

"Now you can go get your calves and put them in for the night. I'll see ya at the house." Before Hugh walked out of the barn, he turned around and said, "Thanks buddy, I couldn't have done it without you."

Jacob winked at his Grandpa, which put another smile on the tired old face.

That evening, as half of the house was already in bed, Eileen decided to call it a night. Before she headed up the stairs, Hugh asked her how the invitations for Thanksgiving were going. There was no light on in the house except for a faint yellow bulb over the stove, but he could see that she was preoccupied with chewing her lip and nervously twisting her auburn hair.

Jacob's turmoil was weighing on her, and she'd forgotten to ask Hugh if he'd talked to him about anything. Now she didn't have the energy, so it would have to wait. She sighed and answered, "Pretty darn good, so far. Everyone I've called says they're coming. Now all I have to figure out is the menu, and where to get a zillion tables and chairs. Maybe I can borrow some from the church. Don't worry, though, I'll figure it out."

"How about you not worrying about that part, sweetie? Jacob and I will be in charge of the seating and of getting the barn ready. Trust me, we can handle it," Hugh assured her.

He wanted more than anything to surprise her and to make her happy. They were a team after all, and it was one of the few ways he could show his appreciation for all that she did.

"Wife is going to supervise the project, we've already talked about it," he said with a wink.

That cracked Eileen up, erasing the shadow of worry on her face. "I think I kind of overdid it with the invites, but I didn't want to leave anyone out, if you know what I mean?"

"Sure, I know what you mean, so don't worry about it. We can handle it. You just focus on the food part, okay? Now let's get some sleep," he said, vanishing into the darkness of the stairs.

Eileen took the steps up to her room two at a time. "I hope I can," she murmured.

SECRETS WE KEEP

"Why didn't you or the office call me, Mary?" Eileen asked Jacob's teacher. She was obviously a little irritated as she stood in the school's main hallway the following morning.

"To be honest with you, Eileen, I forgot all about it," Mary Ashley said. "It was crazy around here yesterday with everyone getting ready for the big football game last night. Apparently, after last week's home game with Pella, a bunch of kids tore up the high school field. A hundred kids from Des Moines, plus their parents, were here for the game. It was all I could do to keep track of our own kids in that chaos."

"I'm awful sorry," she added.

"This morning I made sure that Jacob and Dan were separated, and at least for the time being, everything is fine. They're in gym right now, ignoring each other."

"Please," Mary said, motioning to a closed door, "let's go in here and talk."

When they walked into the small office off the main hallway, the teacher got right to the point. "Do you know Dan, the boy involved?" Mary asked.

"No, I don't. I've never heard his name before yesterday," Eileen said. "But whoever he is, Jacob was pretty mad at him when he got home."

"I don't blame him for being mad," Mary agreed. "I was mad too, but not at Dan or Jacob. I was mad at the whole situation. I hate it when kids fight. I don't know if Dan stole the gloves. He didn't admit to it, and I didn't find them in his locker or in his backpack. I know he doesn't need any because he has his own pair." She sighed and took on a more conversational tone. "Whatever its worth, I'm having Deputy Austen come to school this afternoon, before the bell rings, to talk with Dan; you know, give him a talk about stealing, just in case I'm wrong."

Austen, another lifelong resident of Ottumwa, became a Deputy of Wapello County right out of high school. Eileen knew his parents, and even babysat him a time or two when she was a teenager. Now in his late 20's, single, 6'2" and fit as a fiddle, he looked pretty intimidating, especially in his uniform. That is, until he smiled. When that guy smiled, he became the most beautiful man Eileen had ever seen. Ever. And she wasn't the only one in the county who felt that way. Almost every woman, old or young—unless they were blind—thought the same thing.

Once, Aunt Fara told Eileen, after being pulled over by Austen for driving her tractor down the middle of the highway, that he could pull her over every day for the rest of her life and she wouldn't care.

Part of Austen's beauty was his perfect skin—a bronzy chocolate attributed to his Fox and Sauk heritage. He was a descendant of Chief Wapello himself, for whom the county was named. The young county deputy, the great chief's descendant, was graced with the same facial structures that were carved into the eighteen-foot-tall statue of Chief Wapello located in the town of Agency, a few miles out of Ottumwa.

Mary continued, "I'll do my best to keep those boys separated until this blows over, and I promise that if there are any more problems, I'll call you. No one needs this kind of crap, not you, not me, and certainly not Leila. Do you know Leila Morgan?"

Eileen couldn't place the name. "I don't think so," she said. "Should I?"

Mary stood up to shut the door to the office. Before she went on, she brushed her short faded-blonde hair away, exposing deep worry lines above her almond-shaped eyes. When she sat back down this time, it was on the edge of the chair, closer to Eileen. "She's my sister actually and Dan's mom. She's currently in prison over in Mitchellville."

"Oh, I didn't know!" Eileen gasped. "In prison? What for?"

Mary sighed. "It's a long, sad story. I guess it's no secret, but I'd like it if you kept what I'm about to tell you to yourself, okay?"

"Certainly," Eileen said, noticing tears filling Mary's eyes.

Mary forged ahead. "Leila broke her hip while my brother-in-law, Jud, was in Afghanistan and became addicted to pain pills. She started stealing them from her nursing job, and by the time Jud returned home, she was jobless, living in Comanche with Dan, and shooting up heroin."

Stunned, Eileen blurted out, "Jud? Jud Morgan? I went to school with him. He was always such a shy, sweet guy. Where's he now?"

Clearing her throat, Mary spoke, but barely above a whisper. "Jud killed himself a few years ago, right before Leila was sentenced. I guess he couldn't shake the ugliness of his time in Afghanistan or handle the lack of stability he came home to. I don't really know why he did it, he just cracked, like so many that come home from that senseless war."

"Oh, my God, that poor little boy. So, who's been taking care of him?" Eileen asked.

Mary wiped away her tears, saying, "I have. It's what family does, right? I promised my little sister I would take care of Dan until she got out of prison, and that I will do so for as long as it's needed." As she reached for a tissue. "My sister's a good person, Eileen, a really good person. She just got sucked into a world where you don't have to feel anything. Drugs don't discriminate, they take anybody to hell and back—back only if they're lucky." Mary concluded with a large sigh. "She gets released next week."

"I can't tell by the look on your face if that's a good thing or a bad thing," Eileen said, leaning forward.

"Oh, it's a good thing all right, Leila's been doing so well," Mary said, brightening. "Dan and I have been driving over to Mitchellville every other week for two years, just so they could stay connected. I didn't want either of them to lose faith. That little boy needs his mom, and my sister needs her son."

Mary's face drooped and her attention was lost in the patterns on the office tile floor. It was obvious to Eileen that something else was bothering her, something beyond the drama she'd just revealed. Her sudden silence was torture. It was like reading a story and finding out part of the way through that the rest of the pages were missing.

Eileen broke the spell. "Mary, is there another problem?"

Shaking her head up and down, almost violently, Mary said, "Yes, there's a problem—two in fact. One is that my sister is going to be sent away, yet again, on the day after Thanksgiving. Her release stipulates that she move into a woman's halfway house in Minnesota for eight months. She just told me yesterday. Dan doesn't know it yet. How do you tell a little boy that his mom is going away from him again without that affecting him negatively? I'm so afraid this will undo everything we've worked for over the past two years."

"Oh Mary, I'm so sorry," Eileen cried, but before she could say more, Mary held up her hand.

"The second and most concerning problem I have right now is that I just found out I have breast cancer, which means I also have to go away, at least until spring. I can't take Dan with me while I have surgery, and I'll be no good to him during the months of treatment. So, I'm worried sick. There is no more family, just me. I honestly don't know what to do." Finished at last, Mary looked at Eileen through tears.

Both women sobbed, clutching each other as if to keep from falling off their chairs. And when the crying faded, hiccups took over.

Remembering where and who she was, Mary stood up, wiped her face with the back of her hand, and straightened her blouse and slacks. She was clearly embarrassed that she allowed the dam to break in front of the parent of one of her students.

Without looking at Eileen, she apologized for having poured out her personal life. "I went too far. I wasn't thinking. Once I started talking, it just all came out."

Eileen knew that she couldn't just walk away and go about her life, as if she knew nothing of these people. "I have an idea," she said, squeezing Mary's shoulders, while crumpling the blouse that had just been straightened. "Whatever you do, Mary, don't lose hope. You said it yourself, there's always hope."

Eileen started for the door. "I'll contact you in the next couple days. You just keep those two boys in line. Oh, and don't forget about coming out for Thanksgiving. The boys will just have to put their issues aside. There'll be no fighting on that day. I'll make sure of it, okay?" She waited for Mary's nod, and when it came, she opened the door and walked away.

Outside the school, Eileen sat in her car for a few minutes to pull her wits together, then called Hugh on her cell phone.

TAKING CARE OF THEIR OWN

Hugh was giddy when he answered the phone. Eileen could tell he was in high spirits by his hearty voice and the enthusiastic way he dove right into telling her about a big surprise, but she had to cut him off.

"Sorry to interrupt, but I'm in kind of a hurry. I was just checking in to see if you guys are okay. I was hoping to stop at Sarah's house before I came home. Is that alright? I'd say I'll be about another hour or so?"

"Sure, honey, we're fine," Hugh said. "My 'supervisor' and I just finished up a project in the barn and thought we'd come in for some lunch. Good timing, eh? You go on and tell Sarah we said hello."

"Will do, Hugh. Thanks. I'll see ya soon," she said, hanging up.

Eileen turned off the highway and onto the county road leading to Sarah's house. A large sign reading "Sarah's Stables" stood along the side of the road. In case anyone missed the sign, they wouldn't miss the huge arrow a little farther down the driveway that pointed first time visitors in the right direction.

She was betting on Sarah being home. Eileen knew she gave riding lessons in the afternoons and hoped that it was early enough to get there before the lessons started.

Sarah's driveway was long, typical of old Iowa farmsteads. On each side of the driveway stood huge old oak trees, protecting the ones who traveled there. Those trees were planted long before either she, Sarah, or even their parents were born.

None of Sarah's family wanted to take over the farm after her Grandparents passed away. All her siblings moved away right after high school, and her parents retired to Florida shortly after that. They hadn't understood why their daughter, a young single woman, would choose to live in "that old house."

They tried, to no avail, to encourage Sarah to at least move to Des Moines, where there were more opportunities for someone her age. But Sarah had no desire to flee rural life, and unlike her family, she loved the old farmhouse. It had been built in the mid-1800's by her grandfathers' father, that history alone made it special to her. Except for the lack of insulation, it was perfect.

Over the years, Sarah had the old barn torn down, replacing it with a new, larger, heated one. It housed eight of her horses and six boarders. The barn and tack rooms were packed with saddles and other essential gear, but the part Sarah was most proud of was the spacious and popular riding arena in the center.

She always had a few rescue dogs around the farm, but horses were her life and love. She made her living by giving riding lessons, boarding horses, and breeding horses. Breeding was where her meat and potatoes came from, and though she was just squeaking by, she was comfortable.

Eileen thought of how inviting the old place looked as she parked her car in front of the long, covered porch, generously decorated with pumpkins, gourds, and stalks of corn. Eileen wanted the same warm effect for the Thanksgiving festivities in their barn.

A woman in a red hat was seated in one of several rocking chairs that were placed around the porch. There was a pipe hanging from her thin lips, and she waved at Eileen as she rocked back and forth.

"Hello, Aunt Fara!" Eileen called. *Good* she thought, *Now I can kill two birds with one stone.*

The front door flew open, and two huge Rottweilers came out, wagging their tails as they ran to greet her. In their wake came Sarah, dressed in her usual attire—blue jeans, buffalo plaid flannel shirt, and worn riding boots. A long, brown braid tangled with copper highlights reminded Eileen of a horse's mane hanging over one of the woman's shoulders.

"Hey girl!" Sarah said as she stepped out onto her porch and took a seat in an empty rocker. "I was going to call you tonight to thank you for the Thanksgiving invite. Sounds like a great plan, so count me in. We were just talking about what we should bring. I'm not much of a cook, but I make a mean pecan pie. Any more suggestions?"

"Pie is great. Make seven or eight of them," Eileen said, chuckling. "I should probably be keeping track of what people tell me they're bringing. It's getting confusing. I know Evert said he'd be bringing hams, and Mike's smoking up about ten turkeys. That should cover the meat. Oh, and Pastor Dale said he was going to fry up a ton of chicken livers. That man sure has a thing for chicken livers."

"Yum," Fara said, letting a cloud of smoke—scented with the hint of apple and citrus—escape her mouth. The aroma of tobacco was as inviting as the porch was festive.

"It's going to end up being one big-ass smorgasbord," Eileen said. "So, bring whatever you want. How's that sound for taking me off the hook?" Then, eager to get on with the real reason for her visit, she changed the subject. "Hey, Aunt Fara, I'm glad you're here. I have something I want to ask you—actually both of you."

Fara reached down and picked a handful of walnuts from the basket next to her rocker. "Shoot," she said, shucking one of the oily black balls, exposing the rich nut inside. "I don't hear so good these days, sugar, so come on over here and tell me what's on your mind."

"Yes'm," Eileen said, choosing a chair between the two women.

Fara didn't give the woman a chance to speak before she began, "How's things over at the Roberts?" she asked without looking up from her walnut shucking. "Hugh and Betty okay?" She'd been at the pharmacy that morning and got an earful from the pharmacist about Leroy's experience the Sunday before when he found Hugh and Betty in the road.

"Actually, things are great, Fara. Hugh's acting like a man on a mission now that Jacob's around, and Jacob hasn't quit glowing since we moved out there, thanks in part to you. Hugh loves those calves something awful and, well, there's a light in his eyes that wasn't there before, ya know? I don't know if it's because of Jacob, or because of the animals. All I know is that Hugh doesn't seem as sad as before." Eileen thought about mentioning the bird, Boy, but decided against it. That was too long a story, and she wanted to get to the big reason she came. "Something's different, and in a good way."

"That's great to hear," Sarah chimed in.

"Do either of you know Leila Morgan?" Eileen suddenly asked.

"Of course I do," Fara said. "Known her since she was born, like you girls. Her grandmother and me were pals back in the day. Had a lot of fun too. Why do you ask?"

Eileen smiled. "Who the heck don't you know, Fara?"

"Well, I don't know the President of the United States!"

They all cracked up at that remark, and when laughing died down, Eileen got serious again. "Well, the thing is, I just came from having a meeting with Mary Ashley about some trouble between Jacob and a boy named Dan."

Fara asked, "You mean Dan-The-Man, or some other Dan?"

Astonished, Eileen answered, "Oh, I mean Dan-The-Man all right, but how, may I ask, do you know that he calls himself that?"

The weathered boards under Fara's rocker creaked as she leaned forward wearing a smug look. "'Cause I gave him that name, that's how!"

"Of course you did," she laughed, then turned to Sarah.

"I suppose you know Dan-The-Man too?"

"Sure do," Sarah said. "I've been giving him riding lessons every other Saturday for about a year now, right Fara?"

Fara nodded, "That's right."

It was no secret that Fara paid for just about anything children wanted to learn, particularly if their parents couldn't afford it. It didn't matter what kind of lessons they were: piano, swimming, dance, whatever. It just hadn't occurred to Eileen that riding lessons were a part of that.

"Go on now," Fara said, taking a long draw from her pipe.

"So, you know about Leila being in prison and that her husband killed himself?" Eileen ventured.

Both women looked at each other, nodding in unison.

"Well, how come I didn't know anything about it then?" Eileen asked, feeling out of the loop of common knowledge.

"Sad story, but not all sad stories have sad endings," Fara said. "Mary's been doing a damn good job with that boy, and his mama's going to be getting out real soon. They'll be all right. Now let's hear your question."

"Finally," Eileen said, a bit too loudly. "Since you two seem to know most of what I was going to say, I'm guessing you know the rest of the story too, eh?"

Fara said, "Try me."

"Mary told me not thirty minutes ago that, yes Leila is getting out next week, but that she's being sent away right after Thanksgiving to some halfway house in Minnesota. She'll be gone for another eight months."

Fara's eyebrows raised, confirming this was news to her. Eileen couldn't help but allow the corner of her lip to curl smugly. Being a beat ahead of Fara was a first—and probably a last—so she kept going. "And did you know Mary has breast cancer?"

"Shit!" Fara spat out, throwing a walnut into the yard. "Dammit! Just when those poor folks could see the light at the end of the tunnel, the devil himself turns the light off! Now what's going to happen, did she say?"

"She's scheduled to have surgery in Des Moines soon. She'll have to stay there for her treatment and recovery. That's why I'm here." Eileen continued, "I was kind of hoping that Sarah would consider taking the boy in until either his mom or his Aunt comes home."

Sarah couldn't hide the effect of Eileen's words. The look on her face was sheer horror. "What, me?" she said, faltering slightly. "I don't like kids! You know I don't like kids!"

Both Fara and Eileen smothered a laugh. They knew Sarah preferred animals to most people—everyone knew that—but they also knew most of her clients were children, and she was great with them.

Sarah stood up, pacing the length of the creaky porch. "Tell her Aunt Fara, tell her how I don't like kids. What the heck would I do with a kid anyway? Hell, I'd probably lose him somewhere, or forget to feed him and he'd starve to death, or something. I can't take in a kid," she mumbled. She stopped in front of Eileen. "I'm not the right person for that job, I swear it. An hour or so a day is just about as long as I can handle a kid. To be honest, the idea scares me to death. What about you? You already have one, what's one more, huh?"

Fara and Eileen were still laughing, not really at Sarah, but at how she instantly came unglued at the mere idea of having to take care of a child. It was funny, for sure.

"All I know is that we have to do something," Eileen said. "We can't let that boy go to foster care to live with strangers. Remember, I don't even know who this boy is, so that makes me a stranger. Besides, you both seem to know Dan-The-Man pretty well."

Fara stood up slowly, indicating that she was done with the porch and the dilemma presented on it. It took her a minute to straighten her body, and once she was upright, said, "We're going to do something. And no, we are definitely not going to let him live with strangers." She stuck her pipe in her mouth and lit it again. "I have to think about this." Then, without another word, she stepped off the porch and walked over to her truck, crawled inside, and drove away.

"She's the boss," Sarah said, watching the red hat through the back window as the old pickup bounced down the driveway and disappeared through the tunnel of oaks.

"Yep, she's the boss," Eileen agreed, heading to her own vehicle. When she reached the car, she didn't dare turn around as she called, "Thanks, Sarah. It was fun scaring the hell out of you—well worth the trip out here."

Eileen thought Sarah mumbled something better not heard as the door to the house slammed shut.

DAN~THE~MAN AND JACOB

By the time Eileen got back to the Roberts' farm, a sheriff's cruiser had parked next to the kitchen door. Her heart leapt and dread yanked at her stomach. School wasn't out, she'd just left there an hour before. She prayed that nothing more had happened with the boys. Or worse. Did Betty wander off? Did Hugh have a stroke? Who could've called 911 if Hugh was the one down? *I shouldn't have left for so long,* she thought, unable to keep her mind from jumping to conclusions. What about her parents? They were fine that morning.

If she'd lingered in the car, she'd have puked right there, but she didn't give herself the time, hopping out and running. She would've laid rubber all the way to the house if she had tires on her feet instead of shoes. Hanging onto the counter that divided the kitchen from the dining and living room, she took in the people sitting around the table and asked breathlessly, "What the hell's going on here?"

Jacob, quick on the draw, said, "You shouldn't swear in front of children, mom."

A muffled laugh came from the boy sitting next to him. Eileen guessed that this was Dan-The-Man. He had dimples, a thick tow head of hair, and beautiful teeth—even though one in the front was missing.

"Quiet boy," Hugh said, smacking the top of his grandson's head ever so lightly. "Don't you ever tell your mother what she's supposed to do, ya hear me?"

"Yes, sir," Jacob said, deflated when his attempt to impress Dan-The-Man backfired.

"Everything's all right, honey. We're just having a nice talk with the boys," Hugh said, trying to calm his daughter-in-law but having little effect on her distressed state. "Have a seat."

Eileen crossed her arms to hide her shaking hands. "If you don't mind, I'll stand."

Deputy Sheriff Austen rose and smiled at her. Suddenly, the only thing Eileen could think of was how Fara was missing out. Neither of them wanted to land the deputy for their own—they just enjoyed looking at him.

No crime in looking, she thought, as he started to speak.

"I brought the boys out here in the hope that we could clear some things up. I thought it was better to have this conversation here than at school. Isn't that right, boys?" He looked sternly at the two wide-eyed boys at the table.

"Yes, sir, that's right," Dan-The-Man said, standing as if on cue. He kept his gaze glued to the middle of the table, however, where Jacob's water-resistant winter gloves had been placed neatly.

The boy turned to Eileen. "Mrs. Roberts, I did take— I mean, I stole—Jacob's gloves. It was stupid and I'm sorry I did it. Grandpa Hugh said that as punishment I could work around the farm, if that's okay with you?"

"Grandpa Hugh?" she repeated, glancing over at the old man who quickly looked away. Apparently, he'd handled the situation in her absence.

Eileen didn't answer the kid right away; she wasn't sure where this was going. Instead, she looked over at her son and said, "I want to know what you have to say about this, Jacob."

"In front of these two witnesses," Jacob said, pointing to his Grandpa and the deputy, "I told Dan what you told me about stealing, and how you don't never have to steal unless you're hungry, and I mean really hungry, right? And even then, it's still stealing, but God will forgive you for it because you're starving to death. But not if you're starving to death because you're a lazy bum! I also told him how there's no lower life form than a thief and a liar." Jacob smiled, proud of himself.

Eileen couldn't help but grin. "That's not exactly how I said it, honey, but I'm glad you shared it with him anyway. Do you forgive him, Jacob? Do you think he should be punished for taking your gloves?"

Jacob answered right off. "I think when the deputy came into our classroom and took him away was punishment enough, right Dan?"

Everyone looked to Dan, who was nodding vigorously. "That was pretty embarrassing," he said.

"The rest was kind of cool, mom. Riding out here in a real cop car. I got to sit in the front and 'the fugitive' had to sit in the back." Jacob laughed and so did "the fugitive."

"But do you forgive him?" his mother insisted.

"Yes," Jacob said, "I do."

"Okay then, no more fighting, no more stealing, and furthermore," she said looking right at Dan-The-Man, "no more teaching Jacob 'farm words.'" The last bit nearly made her smile, but she repressed it.

"Do you hear me, Dan?" Eileen asked the boy, whose dimples now vanished as he nodded.

"Yes'm, I promise," he said.

"Then why don't you boys go on outside and let the grownups talk for a while," Eileen suggested.

Not needing to be told twice, the two boys jumped at the chance and quickly disappeared through the kitchen door, slamming it behind them with a bang. The noisy departure woke Betty, and she made a small sound from her chair. Her watery blue eyes searched the room, landing on Deputy Austen.

He nodded and politely greeted her, "How you doin', Mrs. Roberts?"

"Howa Chief," Betty said, raising a hand in greeting.

There was no mistaking what she'd said, and Eileen and Hugh looked at each other with discomfort, the latter quietly getting out of his seat to attend to her.

"Time for a potty break," he said, guiding her away from the chair and into the bathroom, not offering Eileen any assistance in the awkwardness that followed the embarrassing remark.

Eileen didn't know what to say. She was surprised that Betty had responded to Austen at all, but more afraid that the old woman's greeting was something right out of an old western movie—a racial slur.

"Off the wall comments are a symptom of brain deterioration." The words tumbled from Eileen's quaking mouth as she felt the need to explain the components of Betty's disease. "It's quite common at this stage to . . ."

Austen smiled and pointed to the sleeve of his uniform. In big, red embroidery it read, *Chief*. "Don't sweat it, Mrs. Roberts, it's my nickname."

"Thank God," Eileen said, and thought of Fara. She couldn't help but wonder if the old girl had given him his nickname too.

"Being Indian is something I've always been proud of, so when the department said we could add a nickname to our sleeve, I thought, *hell yeah*!" Laughing, he went on, "The Chief Deputy wasn't very happy about there being two *chiefs* in the department, but in the end, he let me get away with it." Pointing to his sleeve again, he said, "The rest is history."

Feeling relieved, Eileen sat down at the table and motioned for Austen to do the same. "What about the boys? Do you think this is the end of the fighting?" she asked.

"Hard to know for sure," Austen said. "But I can tell you they were both pretty scared when I showed up at school today, which is a good thing. It's a knack I have, scaring the hell out of kids. Of course, the uniform and gun on my hip help some. Once we got into my car to head out here, they seemed to forget they were enemies. The goofballs even asked me if I'd take the long way! Hey, want me to give Dan a ride home?"

"No, I think I'll let them hang out for a while. I can drive him home later. I assume Mary knows he's out here?"

"She sure does, but I'll give her a call to let her know you'll be bringing him home later."

"Thank you," Eileen said.

"You know, Mary's pretty strict with that boy," Austen said, as he put on his jacket. "I think kids lie sometimes because the punishment they receive for telling the truth is too severe. It doesn't make it okay to lie, but you know what I mean."

"Yeah, I guess I do," Eileen said, remembering a time when she'd lied to her dad because she was too afraid to tell him the truth. When he found out later, he held it against her for a very long time. Too long, she felt. Such a fine line one walks when disciplining a child with fear. Yep, she did know what he meant.

"So, Austen, have you decided what you're going to do for Thanksgiving?" she asked.

"Thanks for reminding me. I was going to talk to you about that when I got out here, but I forgot. Mom and Dad decided to go to Kansas to spend Thanksgiving with my sisters this year, so I'm free! Count me in. Hey, any chance you invited Sarah?"

"Well, as a matter of fact, I did," Eileen answered with a sly smile. "Why do you ask, hmmm? You have a thing for her?"

"Well, I don't know if I'd call it a *thing*. She's been giving me riding lessons the past few weeks and," he hesitated, well…okay I have a thing for her," he said, blinding her with another gorgeous smile.

"That's great!" she said.

"Now don't you go trying to fix me up. Aunt Fara's already putting her nose in where it don't belong. I've got this, okay?" On his way to the door, he asked, "What would you like me to bring? I hear there's a gob of people coming."

"I think you should call Sarah and ask her what she thinks you should bring," Eileen shot back, grinning.

"Women!" he said, walking out into what was left of the afternoon.

Outside, Dan and Jacob were busy playing tag with the little calves, Bob and Daisy. Dan climbed up on one of the boards circling the pen to catch his breath when he noticed a white picket fence on a hilltop.

"Hey Jacob, what's that over there?" Dan asked, pointing out over the partially snow-covered field.

Running hard, with Daisy right behind him, Jacob reached up with both hands to grab hold of the boards and climbed up next to Dan. Bob was already on the other side of the pen taking advantage of the lack of competition at the feeding trough.

Jacob cranked his head around to where Dan was pointing, then jumped outside of the fence. "It's a graveyard. Wanna meet my family?" he asked in all seriousness.

"Creepy," Dan said, leaping down to catch up. "Why is your family buried out here and not in a real graveyard?"

"This is a real graveyard—it's our graveyard," Jacob replied. "Ain't no strangers buried in there, just our family and some cats and dogs, and I think my dad's bull is there too. Grandpa says it's important to keep your people close to you. That way if you need to talk to them, you can just walk out there and sit down for a visit," he said nonchalantly, kicking snow up into the air with his boot as they walked. "Sometimes I go there just to be alone, other times just to talk."

"Creepy," Dan said again.

When they got to the partitioned, square-shaped segment of farmland, Jacob followed the fresh deer tracks over the little white fence, ignoring the open gate on the other side. He motioned for Dan to follow him as he weaved through the many old headstones, stopping when he came upon a newer, larger one. Pointing, Jacob said, "Dan, meet Charles James Roberts—my dad."

Dan looked down at the stone and then back over to Jacob. "Died in 2006? That's the year I was born, man."

"See the date?" Jacob asked. "That's the day I was born. He died the same day. Never even got to meet him."

Dan felt something he hadn't experienced before. Creepy or not, he realized that the dead had just connected him to the boy standing next to him—the same boy he'd bullied and stolen from. Unconsciously, he moved closer to Jacob, putting his arm around his shoulder. Neither said anything until, out of nowhere, came Boy. The bird landed on Jacob's shoulder, right on top of Dan's fingers.

Dan let out a high-pitched scream and tried to shoo the bird away, which tickled Jacob. But the bird didn't leave. Instead, it hovered just above them until Dan backed away. Then Boy landed once again on Jacob's shoulder.

"Hey, Boy, I've been wondering where the heck you were," he said, watching the bird who looked right back at him.

"You're kidding me, right?" Dan said, putting his hands on top of his head to prevent an unwanted landing or poop bomb.

"Kidding about what? Boy? No, I'm not kidding, he lives here. He lives with the chickens and our cat, Mrs. Nickels. My Grandma saved him after he dive-bombed a window, and now he's part of the family. What's the big deal?"

"But you're talking to . . . to a bird. That's creepy, man!"

Jacob shook his head. "You must like that word, dude, because you've said it like three times already! And there's nothing creepy about it. I talk to all the animals, all the time. What would be creepy is if they talked back to me. But don't worry, so far that hasn't happened," he said as he sat down on the damp ground in front of his dad's grave.

Dan kept an eye on the bird as he took a seat next to Jacob. Then, both boys studied the headstone, each with his own thoughts.

Dan spoke first. "My dad died when I was six. He killed himself."

Jacob jerked his head around to look at Dan.

"Every Memorial Day my Aunt Mary takes me to the graveyard in Comanche where he's buried. She pulls weeds and plants flowers around his grave all day. Sometimes we have a picnic, but usually I just spend the day walking around reading the names on the headstones. I try to memorize as many of the soldiers as I can so when I go back the next time, I can test myself. You know, see if I can find them again. Its huge, that place, with hundreds of soldiers from all different wars buried in there alongside their families. I've made a game out of finding them. My dad was a soldier and . . ." Dan's voice trailed off, mumbling into the wind as he became lost in his thoughts, his story fading away.

Jacob thought about how envious he was that Dan had known his father. He'd known what he looked like, smelled like, and sounded like. But his envy soon turned to empathy, because unlike him, Dan truly knew what he was missing. Right then, Boy left Jacob's shoulder and flew over to Dan's, as if reading his mind.

So, okay, maybe that was a little creepy, Jacob thought.

Dan's trance ended when Boy landed on one of his arms, he had tucked in front him, but this time he didn't scream, or squirm, or try to shoo the bird away. He just turned to face the headstone for Charles James Roberts.

"What do ya say to your dad when you're out here?" Dan asked Jacob.

"Not much, really. Sometimes I tell him about what's going on at school, but lately I've been telling him about the calves, Bob and Daisy. Hey, if I tell you something will you promise not to tell anybody?"

Dan nodded.

"Most of the time when I come out here, it's to cry." Jacob waited for Dan to laugh, and when that didn't happen, he went on. "I don't cry because my dad's out here and not in the house. My mom says it's selfish to cry about that when so many kids don't have no family at all. She says I'm lucky because so many people love me. So, I guess I cry because I can't help it. Sometimes I'm just sad for no reason. Do you ever feel that way?"

Again, Dan nodded, his cheeks pink with cold.

"How about you? You ever talk to your dad?"

"No," Dan answered, thinking about it hard. "I don't know what I'd say to him. 'I miss you. Why did you go away from me? How's the weather down there?' All the things your mom probably thinks are stupid," he said.

Jacob shook his head. "My mom wouldn't think any of that's stupid. You knew your dad, I didn't. You have a right to miss him and maybe even be mad at him for what he did, but then you need to forgive him, so you can be better. Mom says forgiveness is the key to everything in this world. That's why I forgave you for stealing my gloves," he went on, never taking his eyes off his new friend. "Cancer killed my dad, and because of that, I used to be pissed off at God, but I'm not anymore."

"How come?" Dan asked.

"It's that forgiveness thing. I have to believe God has a plan for me. It doesn't mean that the plan is always going to make me happy, but believing it makes things better. I guess that's what ya call faith, dude. Grandpa says that when someone is in your life, it's because God lent them to you for a while. He says they're a gift no matter how long they're with us, and that we should be grateful, no matter what. What do you think?"

Dan furrowed his brow. "I don't know what I think. My Aunt Mary's a Christian, for sure, and probably thinks about things the same way your Grandpa does. We go to the Baptist church downtown. She says that's what I am, a Baptist, but I don't even know what that means," he said, shrugging his shoulders. "Most people in our church are black. My Aunt says black people don't judge a person the same way white people do, and I think she's right, 'cause I remember when we used to go to a different church where everybody was white and they weren't very friendly. They stared at us a lot. My Aunt said they treated us like we were bugs. Next thing I know, boom! We're Baptists and singin' with the black folk."

The boys sat in silence for a minute before Dan spoke again. "My favorite part about goin' to church, besides not being treated like a bug, is the music. It's awesome. Sometimes I swear the walls are going to come down, the way it rocks in there! When everyone is singin' and swayin' to the music is when I feel God the most. It's powerful, man. Want to go with me sometime?"

"Sounds good to me," Jacob answered. "The only music we have at my church is when Mrs. Johnson plays the organ, and it's not something anyone would want to dance to, that's for sure. How about your mom? Is she a Baptist too?"

"No," Dan said. "My mom doesn't go to church, and when I ask her about it, she says that if there is a God, He knows you love Him no matter where you are or what you call yourself. But my aunt makes me go, no matter what my mom says. I think she thinks mom's an atheist."

"What's an atheist?" Jacob asked.

"A person who doesn't believe in God," Dan answered.

"Hmmm, I wonder who she talks to when she's sad or lonely?"

"Don't know, I'll have to ask her that."

"What about your dad?" Jacob asked. "Was he an atheist too?"

"I don't think so, 'cause I remember one time when we were walkin' and found a dead bird in the road. It was a Blue Jay. My dad picked it up and spread its feathers out like a fan. He said, 'Look at these feathers, son. Look at how perfect each one of these polka dots are on them.' I didn't know Blue Jays had polka dots, but they do. Anyway, then he asked me, 'Now, you tell me who else, but God, could've created something so beautifully perfect?' So, yeah, I'd say my dad believed in God."

"Do you live with your aunt because your mom's an atheist?" Jacob asked.

"Hardly," Dan laughed. "I thought everybody knew why I lived with my aunt."

Jacob shook his head.

"Right after my dad died—killed himself—my mom got sent to Mitchellville, a prison for women, because of something she did with pills. We don't talk about it much, except when we talk about drugs and how they'll mess up your life like they did mom's. Me and Aunt Mary go visit her a lot. She's doing real good now." He crossed his fingers and held them up. "She's coming home next week! Just in time for Thanksgiving. I can't wait!"

"Holy crap, man!" Jacob said, feeling like he'd just read a couple chapters from a true crime story. "I guess my mom is right about not feeling sorry for myself. I am lucky! But you're lucky too, Dan. You have your Aunt Mary, your mom, and the Baptists—oh, and me too now!" Jacob added, meaning every word.

Dan's head dipped once as he digested the kind words, then he used his free hand to stroke the small feathers on Boy's head. "I'd like to come out here again sometime and tell you more about my dad, is that okay?"

"You bet! I'd like to know more about him and your mom too." Jacob put a hand on his belly and rubbed it around in a circle. "But all that true-life stuff made me hungry. Let's go to the house and get something to eat."

"Sounds good," Dan agreed.

The boys stood up to begin their walk back through the field, but not before bidding a farewell to the cold stone below them. "See ya later, Dad," Jacob called over his shoulder.

"Yeah, nice to meet ya, Mr. Roberts," Dan said.

Boy simply flew off.

Later that day, when Dan got out of the Roberts' car at his house, he thanked Eileen for letting him come over, not mentioning Deputy Austen or the circumstances that led up to his visit. That was water under the bridge. Before turning to greet his Aunt Mary, Dan said to Jacob, "Thanks dude!" adding two thumbs up.

As they were backing up, Eileen gave Mary a thumbs-up as well. Jacob's mouth dropped open when he realized that Dan's Aunt Mary was his teacher, Ms. Ashley.

Eileen saw the look on Jacob's face. "Small world, isn't it, son?"

"Wow, it sure is."

"And it only gets smaller, honey," she said as they drove down the block and turned off onto the highway.

By the time they got back to the farm, the sun was gone from the sky. They hadn't talked much on the drive home, just idle chitchat and not much of that.

Jacob was eager to get home to his critters, and she'd decided earlier, having watched the boys laugh and talk while inhaling the peanut butter sandwiches she'd made them, to leave the subject of the day alone. All she could do now was hope they'd both learned a lesson. She had no idea the depths of what they learned that day, and it hadn't come from the law or the school but from somewhere deep inside their ten-year-old hearts.

She entered the warm house, thinking about what to make for supper. She was banking on something quick, because she still had so much to do to make sure her Thanksgiving plans were on track. Everyone she had asked was coming, and with only one week to go, she was happy to have the number confirmed. But the size of it was also stressing her out. Thankfully, deciding that everyone would bring something with them, rather than have a set menu, was the best idea she'd had so far. It meant she no longer had to worry about the food, just the seating and decorating the barn.

Hugh had assured her that the tables and chairs were taken care of, an important detail that she hoped was really set, otherwise it would be a disaster. She needed to confirm that with him in a way that wouldn't be insulting or hurtful. He'd seemed so excited to be doing his part, so she would tread lightly, careful not to take that feeling away from him.

The house seemed too quiet when she entered. There was no sign of Hugh or Betty. Even after calling their names from the kitchen, only silence greeted her. The doll lay on the floor by the chair, its painted smile turned halfway toward the carpet. The sight of it sent worry snaking up Eileen's spine.

"Hey, you," Hugh said, the screen door snapping shut behind him.

Eileen spun around to see Hugh and Betty walk arm in arm into the house. Hugh went right to removing his wife's coat, hanging it up in the closet by the door.

"How'd it go?" Hugh asked.

Eileen massaged her collarbone as her heart rate settled, feeling silly she'd gotten such a fright over nothing. "It went fine. The boys seemed okay, even called each other 'dude' a few times and hand bumped like this," she said, taking his free hand and curling it into a fist so she could bump it. "I guess it's something young people do when things are cool between them. I don't really understand it, but it's a good sign. One less thing to worry about." She turned to look in the refrigerator. Now that she didn't have to worry about Hugh and Betty, she could start making supper. "What were you guys up to?" she asked, frigid air wafting over her face.

"We were out in the barn settin' up the tables. Wanted to make sure there were enough, ya know?" Hugh said, leading Betty to the table.

"You got tables and chairs already?" Eileen asked, relieved and surprised.

"Told you we'd handle it, and we did, didn't we, Wife?"

There was no response to his question as he sat her down.

"We have plenty of seats, and plenty of tables too," he said proudly, not offering any information on how he'd come by them. "And that old stove heats the barn up pretty darn good. It should be real toasty on

Thanksgiving. Want any help with supper?" he asked, walking back into the kitchen.

"No thanks," Eileen said, "but if it's okay with you, I think we'll just have soup and sandwiches tonight. I'd kind of like to get going on figuring out the decorations. Then all that will be left to do for Thanksgiving is to eat."

They smiled at each other, then Hugh said, "You don't have to worry about that either. Got that handled too."

"Got what handled?" Eileen asked, pulling out some cold cuts and cheese before shutting the refrigerator door. Her smile was replaced with evident disappointment. Decorating was the one thing she was really looking forward to doing. It was the fun part.

Seeing the look on her face, Hugh said, "I called 'snoopy pants' today, took all I had in me to do it, but I did it. I remembered what a good job she did in the barn for your wedding, so I figured she'd understand when I asked her for any of their leftover pumpkins, and whatever field corn they had, and you know what? She was ecstatic. I guess I don't give that woman enough credit. Anyway, I figured you might want those things for the tables. She even said she'd come out and help if you wanted her to, and maybe bring Patty with her. Did I do right, honey?"

Relieved, Eileen answered, "That's exactly what I was thinking of doing. Thank you, thank you, thank you!"

Her reaction warmed Hugh's heart.

"Do you think you can scavenge up some corn stalks too? I'd love to tie some around the post. And maybe straw bales to for the kids to sit on?"

"Your wish is my command, young lady," he said, bowing grandly. He seemed a little giddy as he went on to ask, "I was going to save this part as a surprise, but what the hell. Guess what else we're going to have out there?"

"I have no idea," Eileen said. "Go ahead. Spill the beans."

"A band, that's what!" he crowed. "Tom called this morning to ask if they could bring the band with them for Thanksgiving. The only catch is that we have to feed the band too, but I told him the more the merrier, right?"

Tom was a pharmacist in Ottumwa, and his wife managed a feed company. In the old days, before children and careers, they hung out with Charly and Eileen, and even played at their wedding as their gift to them. These days, their bluegrass band performed during summer festivals, and played at a few bars in town just for fun—a reprieve from their otherwise intense lives.

Eileen grabbed Hugh around the waist and held on tight, her head pressing against his large chest. "This is going to be the best Thanksgiving ever!" she said.

"That it will," he said, sharing in her excitement.

Now, all she had to do was call Mary, but not to talk to her about the boys' issues or to resolve the dilemma Mary was facing, but to extend her Thanksgiving invitation to Dan and his mother. She was riding on faith that Fara had something in the works by way of a solution for them. She certainly didn't have one. So, she hoped that when she called with the invitation, Mary wouldn't bring it up.

BOY

What a day. I ate, I flew around for a while, then I came home and slept in the sun with the furry one. Then I followed the little guys into the field down by the river and hung out with them for a while.

Then it was home to eat some more. Yep, life is pretty darn good.

THE QUESTIONS KIDS ASK

Jacob entered the kitchen, whistling. By this time, Hugh and Eileen sat at the table with Betty working on their supper.

"Take your shoes off and come and eat," his mother said.

"Be right there, mom," he answered.

Jacob sat down, diving right into his sandwich. Mouth full, he asked no one in particular, "Did you know that Dan-The-Man doesn't have a dad either?"

"Please don't talk with food in your mouth, it's gross," his mother said rather than answering his question.

It was Hugh who answered him. "Yes, I knew that son. I remember when it happened. It was a terrible thing for sure, a sad time for many people, especially for his son. Dan's daddy's head was never right after being in the war. He just couldn't get back to livin' once he came home. It's a sickness that some veterans have. I think it's called PTSD."

Jacob quit chewing so he could hear better, listening intently to his Grandpa. He asked, "Do you think God forgives a person for killing themselves?"

"Sure I do," Hugh answered. "That's what God does, forgives. It's too bad people don't do the same," he mumbled, not mentioning how he believed that they might not get through the gates of heaven.

Eileen cleared her throat and jumped in before Hugh started in with a rant about hypocrisy. "Sounds like you and Dan-The-Man have something in common," she said.

"We do, in a way. I mean, both of us lost our dad. But he knew his and I didn't," Jacob said, pointedly.

"That's not what matters, honey," Eileen said. "What matters is that you both lost someone you loved, and that loved you. That's a big deal, and now it's something you and Dan share. I hope you guys can talk about that someday."

"Oh, we did. Today. I took him to the field to meet dad, and one thing just led to the other, as you say." Satisfied, Jacob started to stuff his mouth again.

Eileen and Hugh smiled at the boy, waiting for more on the subject, but it appeared that was the end of it for the time being.

"I'm going to call his aunt tonight and make sure she knows that Dan is welcome to come here for Thanksgiving. His mom too," Eileen said then.

"Yeah, I wanna meet her. Did you know she's in prison? And she's an atheist too? I never met an atheist before," Jacob said matter-of-factly, downing the last of his milk.

"Okey-dokey then," was all Eileen could say to that, relieved, but also surprised that he was more interested in someone being an atheist than being in prison. "Anybody want a bowl of ice cream?"

That night, when everyone disappeared into their rooms, Eileen began picking up around the living room, noticing for the second time that day that the doll lay forgotten on the floor beside Betty's large leather chair. As she picked it up, Eileen wondered if Betty's time with her doll, Boy, had come and gone. She placed it in the chair anyway, covering all but its worn cloth head with the afghan.

"Time will tell," she said aloud, turning off the last of the lights, then following the moon's shadow towards the stairway. Climbing between her cold sheets, Eileen remembered the day her mother brought that very doll home for her and how she'd loved it right off. She chuckled to herself, remembering how she'd named it Lisa, after her best friend who moved away when they were in first grade.

Back then, the painted-on eyes were fresh and blue, and the lips were a bright cherry red, the color of ripe fruit right before it falls away from the stem. Her mother bought it from a woman who made and sold craft items to benefit their church. Eileen was glad now that she'd kept it, glad that it still had a purpose and was loved, if even only for a short time.

Then her thoughts drifted to Mary. She'd been so upbeat during their brief phone conversation, given the circumstances facing her. *Tough lady*, she said to herself. After she turned off the light, she said a little prayer— not to God, but to Aunt Fara.

A MAN CALLED CHOD

The next morning, Hugh got up early and dressed Betty in extra warm clothes so they could head outside and catch Eliza before she was finished collecting their eggs. He usually avoided this encounter, but now he sought it. He wanted to secure the things Eileen wanted for the decorations, so there would be little left for her to do but enjoy herself. Truth was, he was excited to finally let her see what he'd done to the barn. *Soon*, he thought.

Eileen was also up by then, groggy and in her pajamas, but up. She didn't question Hugh when they went outside so early. Jacob had another hour before he had to get up and get ready for school, so she drank up the silence of the house.

Pouring a cup of coffee, she sat down to muster up the courage to call Fara. That required a couple cups of the coal-black liquid. Her curiosity about what was going to happen to Dan-The-Man was driving her nuts. She cared about the fate of this boy and his poor aunt, and now with Leila coming home in less than a week, she could only hope Fara would come through. At last, she put down her cup and picked up the phone.

After many rings, a deep voice answered, "Y'ellow?"

Surprised that someone other than Fara answered the phone, it took a few seconds for Eileen to answer. "Morning, this is Eileen Roberts calling. I was wondering if Fara was up and around yet?"

The question brought a deep chuckle from the other end of the line. "Hello Eileen Roberts, this is Chod. Just happened to hear her phone ringing and ran inside. Didn't mean to throw you off. She's up all right, but long gone, kid."

"Gone already?" Eileen said, surprised. "Would you mind giving me her cell phone number? I need to ask her something."

Another chuckle came through the line. "Cell phone? Fara doesn't have a cell phone," Chod said, clearly amused. "But if you want, I can leave her a message and have her call ya back when she gets home. You know, like we used to do in the old days?"

Eileen was amused, but also frustrated. "That'd be fine, thank you. Hey, you don't happen to know where she went do you?" she added quickly.

"Sure do, she went over to Mitchellville to pay a visit to Leila Morgan. Plans on being back here after lunch. Everything okay over there?"

"Yeah, everything's fine, Chod, thanks for asking. I just wanted to ask her something, but I guess it'll have to wait. Have a good day and see ya soon."

"Lookin' forward to it, Eileen. Tell Hugh and Betty hello for me," he said as he hung up.

Fara must have something up her sleeve or she wouldn't drive all the way over to Mitchellville, Eileen thought. It's not that she'd doubted Fara when she said something would be done, it's just now she had to wait to find out what that something was, and how she could help.

GRACE COMES IN UNEXPECTED PACKAGES

Already dressed and raring to go, Jacob appeared at Eileen's side just as she rang off with Chod. "Morning, honey," she said. "Seems everybody's up early today. How about some scrambled eggs and cinnamon toast for breakfast?"

"Sounds good, but give me fifteen minutes, okay? I want to go see dad really quick, and then check in on the girls." He patted his mom on the back as he slipped into his boots and rushed out of the house in a hurry.

"Strange," Eileen murmured to herself. "Things surely are getting stranger and stranger around here." She laughed and went to make breakfast.

Jacob passed by the open door to the chicken coop where he saw three people were crammed inside.

"Morning all," he said without stopping to ask what they were doing in there. He skipped all the way down the lane, passing the barn, then the stock yard, and setting off into the field, following the same tracks he and Dan made the day before.

Arriving at the silent headstone bearing his father's name, he said, "Hey dad, I just wanted to say thanks for yesterday. Your being here really helped out my friend." Jacob stood with his hands in his pockets for a couple minutes before adding, "Well, that's all I wanted to say for now. Got to get ready for school. Love ya." Then he took off, running towards the barn to let his girls out.

On his way back to the house, he noticed the door to the coop was closed and the three crooked bodies now stood in the driveway talking. He watched his Grandpa hug Mrs. Reeve, making Jacob wonder if that made his Grandma, the third one of the group, jealous. He let out a puzzled grunt as he slammed into the kitchen.

"What's that noise all about?" his mom asked.

He slipped off his boots and said, "Adults are goofy." He was quick to dive into his breakfast. "This is really good. Thanks, mom."

"You're welcome, son, I'm glad you like it. Hey, I'm goin' over to Grandma and Grandpa Erickson's today. Got any messages for them?"

"Yeah, tell them I can't wait to see them on Thanksgiving, okay?"

"You bet," she said, sitting down beside him to finish yet another cup of coffee.

Eliza was gone by the time Eileen and Jacob left the house. Hugh stood at the back of his truck, assessing the contents of its bed, when the two walked up. He leaned against the open tailgate where Betty sat, dangling her legs. He was no doubt protecting her from falling off. She wore his coat on top of hers, a hat, and the familiar blank stare.

It didn't matter to Eileen or Jacob that she didn't look their way or acknowledge their approach. All that mattered to people who loved her was that she was safe and content, and she was clearly both. The skinny legs that rocked over the tailgate with ease confirmed it.

"What's up, you two?" Eileen asked, walking towards her car.

"Talked to Eliza this morning, and she said we could go over anytime to pick up the things you asked for," Hugh answered. Patting his wife on the leg, and looking up at the sky, he added, "I thought today would be a good day for a drive, but first I have to clean out some of this junk." He pointed to the back of his truck. "Sure would like to get it all in one load."

"That's awesome, Hugh, thanks a ton. Breakfast is on the table and I'll be home around noon. I'm goin' over to mom and dad's for a while. You two be careful," she said, feeling concerned. She knew they hadn't been away from the farm in quite a while, but she also knew her place, and it wasn't to give this man advice or lecture him about being careful. The pecking order hadn't changed just because she was living there. Hugh was her elder and the man of the house. She would always be respectful of that.

"Bye, Grandpa, bye Grandma," Jacob said, closing the car door behind him, and off they went.

Fara had been at Mitchellville for less than an hour before she and Leila came up with a plan for Dan-The-Man's immediate future. With her job there finished, they hugged, and Leila was led away from the visitor's room by a friendly female guard. Fara noticed how easily the guard and Leila talked as they disappeared through a large steel doorway. They seemed more like friends than prisoner and guard.

Fara turned towards the exit door meant for visitors, but as she made her way towards it, a tough looking inmate in a white t-shirt and prison-issued orange pants leaned against the wall, giving Fara the once over.

"I need a cigarette," the woman barked.

"Yeah, and people in hell need ice water too," Fara said, never missing a step as she passed the inmate and guard, the latter of whose face broke into a large smile.

"Amen, sister," the guard said to Fara's back as she locked the door behind her.

Back in Ottumwa, Eileen arrived to find her dad busy playing bridge in the Silver Woods great room. "Hey sugar," he said, looking up when she took a place at his side.

After her dad proudly introduced his daughter to the other guys at the table, she kissed his head, said "Good luck," then made her way down the pastel-colored hallway to her parents' unit.

Inside her parent's new digs, Eileen sat admiring the way her mother had made the small space look like home. Her mother busied herself in the kitchenette making coffee. Not that Eileen needed any more coffee, but she wasn't going to be a party pooper and spoil her mom's good intentions.

Eileen was so glad that her parents seemed settled and content in their new surroundings. It was a load off her shoulders, which she knew had been part of their plan, even if they wouldn't admit to it. She loved them for that, and for so many thousands of other reasons.

"What are your plans for tomorrow, mom?" she asked.

Standing at the counter in her red mock-velvet running suit with matching lipstick, her mother asked, "Why, what's up hon?"

"I just thought you might want to come out and help me decorate the barn. It'll be fun, just you and me. Dad can come too if he wants, but there isn't going to be any job for him to do."

"That's perfect, because he doesn't want a job," Katherine said, chuckling. "He can visit with Hugh, though. How's Betty doing?"

"That's a hard one to answer," Eileen sighed. "She's doing all right, considering. However, I think she's moved into another stage of her dementia."

"What does that mean, a 'stage'?" Katherine asked.

Eileen explained. "Like with Alzheimer's, in the beginning a person begins to lose details, dates, names, appointments, and so on. Then, as the disease progresses and consumes more of their short-term memory, what's left are mostly memories of long ago—like childhood—and only fragments at that. The medical world calls the progression 'stages,' which gives us some idea of what's next, and what to expect. It's never good. It takes years sometimes for those around them to notice what's happening, because we assume forgetting is a normal thing for someone getting older. Imagine all the people living alone that have no family at all, or no family active in their daily lives. Think how long they suffer before any intervention takes place."

"Try to imagine, mom," Eileen said, with tears in her eyes, "walking outside of your house and becoming lost in your own front yard. Some people wander off and are never found because no one knows they're missing. And they can't call anyone because they don't remember anyone to call."

Katherine shuddered.

"Betty's been lost many times, but so far, Hugh's always found her. He dresses her, takes her to the bathroom, wipes her butt, feeds her, and so on. He's been doing all of this for a very long time, all by himself. He's familiar to her, only because he's been the constant presence in her life, not because she knows who he is. Having someone familiar is no small thing in that strange world." Eileen couldn't stop once she got going. "She doesn't know me or Jacob, and we don't care. Jacob's so smart, mom. He treats her no differently than he always has. I think it's safe to say that Betty's in the late stages of dementia, which means soon she won't be able to function at all. We just started pureeing her food so she doesn't choke, because she doesn't remember how to swallow. I think we moved out there at just the right time. Hugh needs my help."

"You're awfully sweet, ya know that?" her mom said, smiling at her daughter.

"It's all sweet," Eileen said, "but also sad at the same time. I wish I could tell you some of the things that happen around there, but I wouldn't do them justice if I tried. Just believe me when I say that every now and then, a small miracle takes place. Betty goes from saying nothing for days, then all of a sudden, she'll say one word or do one thing and we all understand its meaning. That little bit of something tickles us and makes Hugh so happy. He's changed a great deal in the past few weeks. It's amazing to watch."

"What's wonderful, honey, is how powerful and important love is," Katherine said. "I think that's why some of us old people get older faster and fade away quicker. I've seen it happen to people I've known my whole life. There's nothing to keep 'em going. That's why they say animals make such a difference in older people's lives. They're something to love and be loved. It's a proven fact! I'm so darn proud of you, Eileen. Charly would be too."

"Thanks mom, I think he would," she said, taking one last sip of coffee. But mid-sip, Eileen's phone rang, interrupting their conversation. She looked at the caller ID. *Kremer*. "Excuse me, I'm expecting this call," she said as she got up from the table and went to the couch.

"Hello?" Eileen answered.

"Y'ellow," came the same deep voice as before. "Eileen?"

"Yes, this is Eileen. Is this Chod?"

"How'd ya know it was me?" he asked, surprised.

"I'm psychic," Eileen declared, not feeling the need to explain caller ID or that his way of greeting had tipped her off. "What's up, Chod, Fara back yet?"

"She is, and she asked me to call you, so you don't fret. Those were her exact words. 'Don't fret.' Said you'd know what she was gettin' at. Anyway, I was calling to ask you if your boy could come to the ranch after school to help me and Dude out with some new calves? Already asked Mary if her nephew could come out too. I'd be happy to pick him up at school if it's okay. We'll feed him when we're done and bring him home before it's too late. Whaddya think?"

"Well, it's kind of short notice, but I guess it's okay. I'll call the school and let them know you'll be picking him up. Don't have him out too late, ya hear?" she added.

"Got it, and thanks, kid," he said, hanging up without saying goodbye.

During the call, Katherine motioned to Eileen that she would be right back and left the unit to check on the guys. Eileen stayed seated on the couch with its noisy plastic covered cushions and waited for her mother to return, all the while wondering what was up with the Kremers. They had never asked Jacob to their ranch before. Something was going on, all right; she was sure of it. She was also pretty darn sure that Aunt Fara was behind whatever it was.

With Jacob working after school, she figured she might as well take advantage of the free time it afforded. So, she decided that after visiting her mother, she'd stop by Sarah's place. There was something she wanted to find out from her too.

As Eileen turned into Sarah's long driveway, she noticed how the morning's blue sky was quickly clouding over, disguising the time of day. Snow threatened, and she kicked herself for not bringing a jacket along. She was just about to get out of her car when she caught movement out of the corner of her eye.

She saw two riders on horses way across the pasture, both with long flowing hair that danced up and down as they rode. At first it looked like two women, but after a few minutes she recognized Deputy Austen and Sarah.

She'd never seen Austen without a hat on, except for when he was a little kid. Back then, everything about him was short, hair included.

She laughed out loud, remembering what a funny kid he'd been, always pulling pranks of one kind or another on her when she babysat. He was gifted with a sense of humor, something Eileen didn't believe could be taught or bought, like common sense. It was something a person was either born with or without, and Austen had both. As far as she was concerned, he was perfect for Sarah.

She watched as the two rode fast and hard, maneuvering around and around each other, as only experienced riders could. They reminded her of skilled barrel racing events at the rodeos. She sat in her car for about ten minutes, enjoying the show without their knowledge, before it hit her.

"Riding lessons, my ass. You sly dog, Austen," she mumbled out loud.

Eileen had come out there to snoop, with the main goal of setting them up if possible. But they'd beaten her to the punch. It was obvious they had a thing for each other, something she could plainly see from her car.

She felt like a window peeper, but she couldn't have been happier. As she headed home, she wondered whether old Eliza wasn't the only one deserving of the name "snoopy pants."

Feeling awkward and nervous, Chod and Dude walked into Hoak Elementary school together to retrieve the boys they'd been sent to pick up. They stood outside the office doors, having left their names with the school secretary. She looked them up and down suspiciously when they told her who they were there to pick up, even making them show their driver's licenses to prove who they were.

When the bell rang, what looked like a swarm of miniature people came running from all directions, some heading for the same door where the big men waited patiently.

Dude said to Chod, "I feel like a giant in here."

"In that green coverall you're wearin' I'd say you look like the Jolly Green Giant," Chod shot back.

They chuckled as their eyes flicked over the hordes of children running by them. Out of the stampede, two young boys appeared, wearing grins as wide as the Raccoon River.

"Ready to roll?" Chod asked the boys.

"You bet we are, sir," Dan-The-Man answered.

"Let's hit it!" Jacob added, without hesitation.

The secretary watched through the window as the four climbed into the large blue diesel truck, writing the license plate numbers down before it pulled away, just in case.

Ten minutes later, Mary walked into the office and checked the sign out sheet. She smiled to herself as she read the names. She stayed away from their rendezvous spot on purpose, even though it was a hard thing for her to do. She was controlling and she knew it. She'd even admit that maybe she was a little too strict with her nephew, but she loved him so. All she'd ever meant to do was protect him.

Now, she was losing control. Their lives were taking a turn not of her choosing, and she knew that she had to have faith and trust in those around her.

When Fara called that morning to ask her if it was okay if Dan came out to the ranch after school, she'd also kindly reminded her that not everything was hers to decide. She suggested holding off telling Dan about his mother having to leave again and to wait for Leila to come home so that she could talk to her son first.

Before Fara said goodbye, she assured Mary that things would work out. Fara had a way of reassuring a person, for which Mary was more than grateful. As hard as it was for her to not be in control of everything, she was taking Fara's advice, even admitting to herself that not being in control was a welcomed relief.

Dan had been so excited when she told him the Kremers needed a ranch hand, and that they wanted to give him a shot at it. He needed men in his life, good men, and if he happened to learn how to work hard in the process, that would be icing on the cake.

It was time for Mary to go home, and with Dan away for dinner, maybe even run a hot bath and drink a glass of wine. It was time for her to let go and worry about herself for a change.

Snow had begun to fall by the time Eileen arrived back at the farm. The rooftops were covered in white, as were the vast open fields. The heavy, wet snow clung to random boards on the buildings and gray smoke billowed and curled its way out of the barn's chimney, reminding her of a picture-perfect Christmas card.

Eileen smiled, thinking how Hugh was always one step ahead of her. The smoke and the four-wheeler tracks that were slowly being erased by the snow gave him away.

She followed the tracks to the barn and entered slowly and quietly through the large doors. It was warm and toasty inside, just like Hugh had said it would be. He was on the opposite end of the barn near the stove, stacking firewood into a neat pile while Betty sat close by on a bale of straw, watching him. They hadn't noticed her yet, so she hung a left to say hello to the bedded calves. When she turned back around, she almost tripped over the pumpkins piled into one of the vacant stalls, and next to that pile was another one of corn stalks and random varieties of squash in all the colors of autumn.

At that moment, Eileen didn't think life could get any better than it was—that is, until she rounded the posts by the stalls and faced the center of the barn. There, four beautiful pine tables stood with matching benches tucked underneath. The tables were long and narrow, designed to seat many. They reminded her of the family tables she'd seen in a few Amish homes.

There would be no wobbly pop-up tables and no folding chairs to separate guests from one another during their Thanksgiving feast. Her guests would sit shoulder to shoulder as they talked, and ate, and drank, until the only thing left for them to do was dance.

A squeal of delight came from deep within her, making Hugh jump and turn away from the woodpile. Betty never flinched.

With open arms, he yelled to Eileen, "Surprise!" His deep voice sent echoes throughout the large space, like a stone being skipped across water.

Eileen came running to him like a child, landing right in his arms. "I love it! I love it! I love it!" she cried.

Only then did Betty look away from the pile of firewood, and with no one watching she stood up and shuffled through the tangled straw and dirt to where the two stood and joined them in a group hug.

"Yep, it doesn't get any better than this," Eileen said, her voice muffled by shoulders and coats as she hugged them tightly.

BOY

When the weather turned nasty, I decided to head inside. My buddies were already there, taking up all the available nests, which meant I wouldn't be sleeping alone. Again.

I wasn't complaining, it's just that sleeping lightly to avoid being smooshed gets old.

Anyway, so there I was, perched up high and minding my own business while I dried off my feathers. The only noise other than a coo or two was the furry one, crawling around under our house—hunting, I assumed—when all of a sudden, out of the corner of my eye, I saw something come in through MY hole in the wall!

I teetered, almost falling off my perch. For a moment I thought I'd been wrong and maybe it wasn't the furry one I heard under the house, but the boogeyman.

I've heard stories about the ruthless weasel that kills whatever it can, but so far, I've been lucky. I haven't seen him around. The others told me how he steals their eggs when they're not looking.

Rotten, rotten boogeyman!

And then I saw her. It wasn't the boogeyman making noise, not at all. It was someone that looked a lot like me, but prettier.

She came in through my hole and landed on the windowsill next to my stash of seed, shaking the wet snow from her beautiful brown body.

Trust me, I didn't mind. And if you could've seen her, you wouldn't have minded either.

FARM HAND

Chod stood in the middle of one of the many rutted roads on the ranch, looking out over his new employees in the distance. He waved both arms to get their attention. "Time to go, you can stop now!" he yelled at them, with no visible effect on either of the boys.

Once they'd finished shoveling manure out of one of the barns, Dude promoted them to dumping feed in the troughs along the fence line. The allure of driving a small tractor around made the slow, grueling work seem worth it. The boys were oblivious to anything other than whose turn it was to drive, so the cattle were lining up faster than they could drop the feed.

Dude had expected as much. He knew he'd be the one to finish up after they'd left, which was fine by him.

Both men were surprised at how much they enjoyed the boys' company; they had no expectations when they picked them up from school a few hours before. The mission for the day, which they would soon be sharing with Fara, was accomplished.

Chod jumped in his Ranger and headed down to where the tractor crept along the side of the road. The two boys didn't even look over when he pulled up beside them.

"Hey!" Chod called out, startling them, but definitely getting their attention. "Time to go, boys. I promised everyone we'd have you home early, and I intend to keep that promise. I don't wanna make anyone mad on your first day of work, now turn the tractor around and park it alongside the pole barn where ya got it, ya hear?"

"Yes, sir," they answered in unison.

Chod pulled away, watching them from the rear-view mirror. He chuckled when he saw them instantly begin Rock Paper Scissors to determine who got to drive the tractor back to the barn. It was a game he remembered from his own childhood, and it tickled him to know that it wasn't obsolete, like so many other things.

Jacob must have won, because Chod saw him grab hold of the steering wheel before Dan's butt even cleared the seat.

When Dan and Jacob got home from work that night they smelled like shit—literally. But each wore a smile that no one could've stolen away.

Independently, and at their own homes, the first question out of their mouths was, "When can I work again?"

Eileen was thrilled that her son was so excited, because it meant that the boys were getting along. She was certain that Mary felt the same way, but with Thanksgiving now only three days away, Eileen decided "work" was going to have to wait until the long holiday weekend. That didn't please Jacob, nor did it shut him up. She listened from the kitchen as Jacob told his grandpa about how he got to drive a tractor, and when she butted in to object to someone his age driving anything with a motor in it, Hugh held up his hand to quiet her. Frustrated, but noticing the serious look on his face, she heard him out.

"I was driving a truck 'round this farm when I was his age. Course I couldn't drive it on the road, but around the farm was okay. That's how I learned to drive. I think I was seven or eight, even younger than Jacob. This boy has to learn sometime, honey, because I'm counting on him to help me out in the fields this spring."

Jacob sat next to his grandpa, nodding his head in agreement. There was no arguing with them, not now anyway, so Eileen shut right up, making the motion of buttoning her lips, which made them smile. She would take the subject up with Dude and Chod later, before Jacob's next "job."

At the Ashley home, things were very much the same, except that when Dan asked when he could work again, his aunt said, "Tomorrow's fine. The guys will pick you up from school, just like they did today. Now go git in the shower and wash that crap off of you!"

Dan looked up at Mary, his face filthy, eyes sincere. "Thanks, Aunt Mary, for everything you do for me." Then he scooted down the hall to wash up.

Mary had waited a long time to hear those words but hadn't figured she'd hear them until he grew into a man and reflected on the time they'd spent together. Now, she only hoped she would live long enough to see him become a man.

Mary was happy with the plan Fara had in store for Dan. It was certainly better than anything she'd thought up, which was no plan at all. He would go out to the Kremer ranch every day but Thanksgiving. His mom would be home soon, and she could talk to him about the next eight months. Hopefully, by then he would be open to moving to the ranch to live with Chod and Dude, at least until his mom came home for good, or until she came home from Des Moines. She crossed her fingers and even looked down at them for extra luck before she warmed Dan's supper.

Hugh fed the calves for Jacob and reminded him during supper that his new job couldn't get in the way of his chores. Jacob said he understood and thanked his grandpa for feeding them just this once.

After he was done eating, he wanted to say hello and goodnight to his critters. "I'll be right back, mom," he said, heading outside with a flashlight.

"I guess it's time for bed," Hugh said to his wife, who was already fast asleep in her chair.

Before he got up from the table, Eileen remembered to tell him that her parents would be coming over in the morning. She was excited to begin the decorating. So much so, that she really didn't care who helped her. The barn was going to be perfect, no matter what, thanks to Hugh.

"That'll be just fine, honey. Haven't seen them in a while. Your dad has always got a few good stories to tell, and I've been saving up my BS for months." With a chuckle, he turned to his wife. "Okay then, woman, let's go on to bed. You got a big day tomorrow."

Betty woke up as he lifted her from the chair, and as he did, he looked around for her baby, but it was nowhere to be found. So be it, as long as she wasn't missing him, he decided to let it go.

Eileen watched them enter the bathroom and heard the facet squeak. Over the sound of water, she swore she heard laughter, but then Jacob came running in, pulling her attention away from the bathroom and whatever private joke that was going on inside of it.

"I see you've found your surprise, mom," Jacob said, pulling off his dirty clothes at the door until he had nothing left on but his Incredible Hulk underwear.

"I sure did, and I hear you had something to do with it," she smiled.

Jacob walked over to his mom at the table and put his arms around her neck. "We wanted to make you happy, and I'm sooooo glad it worked!" he said.

When he released his grip on her, she kissed his cheek. "It worked all right. Now, as soon as the bathroom's free, I want you to get cleaned up. You stink!" she scolded with a grin.

"Dang," he said, walking into his bedroom.

The next day, the boys bragged to their classmates, and anyone else that would listen, about having driven a tractor at their "job." Some of the kids didn't believe them, which made the story grow and morph into more than it had been, and though they shared in the notoriety they were creating, Jacob couldn't help but be jealous that Dan was getting to go to work that day without him.

He envisioned Dan driving the tractor around all by himself but tried not to show his annoyance. To deal with it, he flirted with Kary Lynn, a classmate that Dan had a crush on.

Flirting at this age only meant he teased her about whatever a kid could think of—which wasn't much—but in this case, Dan took notice.

Lucky for the kids, a substitute teacher happened to be in the classroom that day, and as everyone knows, no matter the era, the unspoken rule is that you can take advantage of subs. And they did. Some kids talked back and forth from desk to desk, while others milled around the room, as if the teacher were invisible.

Dan interrupted Jacob's conversation with Kary Lynn, shouting from across the room and trying with what little he had to steal her attention away from his new friend.

"Hey, Kary Lynn, what are you doin' for Thanksgiving?" he called out.

Kary Lynn flipped her long blonde hair from side to side, loving the double attention. "I'm going to the Roberts' farm with my family," she answered.

Both boys looked at each other in surprise, and before either of them could say anything, Beth, who was on the other side of the room, piped in, "I'll be there too!"

Beth was a little girl with brown curly hair and big brown eyes to match. She had shown interest in Jacob before, which until that moment he couldn't have cared less about. Girls were still gross in his opinion, but for some reason the look she gave him made him warm all over. He wondered what the heck was happening to him as he moved away from Kary Lynn and walked across the room to Brown Eyes.

In no time, Kary Lynn and Dan followed him over. The four kids huddled together like they were members of some prestigious Thanksgiving club. Kary Lynn attempted to one-up the rest of them by talking about how her parent's band was going to be the entertainment for the festivities.

A boy named Peter, or Booger Eater as he was known since kindergarten, interrupted. Smugly scooting his chair over to the group, he said, "Hey, my family's coming too! My mom's the fiddle player and everyone knows you can't have a bluegrass band without a fiddle player."

Kary Lynn had been trumped. She rolled her eyes at Booger Eater but left the subject of who was the most valued band member alone. She didn't want to argue, only brag.

Jacob thought about adding his two cents but decided against it, noticing how Beth seemed disinterested in a pissing contest. He liked her more because she didn't want to participate.

Dan did want to jump in to tell everyone about his mother coming home and how she would be at the Roberts' farm for Thanksgiving, just like everyone else. But an unfamiliar apprehension stopped him. For the first time, it crossed Dan's mind that others might have questions or opinions about his mother, and he was in no mood to hear them. He would, however, defend her tooth and nail, if and when the time came.

The kids talked on about music and dancing, and how they planned to eat until they were sick. Then the bell rang, emptying the room out like magic.

Dan was eager to see Chod and Dude again, but he also knew that it bothered Jacob that he got to go to work without him. For the first time in his life, he had a true friend, and he didn't want a dumb tractor to come between them. So, he jogged down the hallway and caught Jacob at his locker.

"Hey dude, don't worry. Friday, you can drive the tractor all day if you want. And just for you, I'll shovel the shit."

Jacob's face lit up. *Girls smirls*, he thought as he bumped Dan's fist. Friends were way better. "Thanks," he said. And he meant it.

When Dan arrived with Chod and Dude that day, they passed a young boy on a tractor, the same tractor Dan and Jacob drove the day before. Dan jerked his head towards the back window and asked, "Who's that?"

"That's John Ray, he works out here sometimes," Dude said as he drove the big truck up the dirt road.

"He looks like a Mexican. Mr. Thompson down at the 7-Eleven says Mexicans are lazy," Dan said, watching the kid dump feed along the fence line like a pro.

Dude didn't respond to Dan's comment, but Chod, sitting in the passenger seat, did. "We have a few Mexicans working here, and I got to tell ya, son, they're some of the hardest workers we have. Whaddya think of that?"

"I'm not sure what to think about that," he answered, as honestly as a ten-year-old could.

"Many of the Mexicans round here are migrant workers," Chod went on. "Know what a migrant worker is, Dan?"

"No," the boy answered, turning away from the window to face the back of the men's heads in the front seat.

"A migrant worker is someone who follows the seasons of crops, picking fruit and vegetables mainly. They hand pick the crops, which is grueling work. Sometimes entire families work in the fields together, harvesting a crop of one kind or another, and the majority of them just happen to be Mexican," Chod said.

Dude added, "There's a town few hundred miles from here called Muscatine, known for its musk melons. Know who the majority are that live in that town, boy? Mexicans, that's who. And why is that? Because a long time ago, they migrated there to pick melons and other things. Many of them stayed and made it their home."

Dude went on to explain that migrant workers travel from state to state, crop to crop, working long hours in the hot sun for wages most other people are "too good" to work for.

"Hell, do you know if it wasn't for Mexicans, we wouldn't have fruit or vegetables in our markets?"

"What are you saying? That white people are lazy?" Dan asked in all sincerity.

Deep laughter came from the front seat, from both men.

"No, that's not at all what I'm saying," Dude said. "Lazy comes in all colors. What I am saying is that most people—okay, a lot of people—are too proud to work for low wages. It just turns out that a lot of those folks are white. Pride can be a funny thing, boy. And I don't mean ha-ha funny. Some folks' pride comes from being able to support their families, even if it means they have to work more than one job to do it. While others think they're too good to work those same jobs. Instead, they sit on their butts and collect welfare. Tell me, where's the pride in that, boy?"

Feeling like the conversation might be getting too deep for a ten-year-old, Chod butted in. "Okay, okay, the bottom line is this: If you're a hard worker, you might not have the newest cars or the latest fashion, but you'll have self-respect, and in our opinion, that's something to be proud of. Now on that note, let's get to work!"

The three of them climbed out of the truck as soon as it came a stop and headed to the main barn so Dan could change into his work clothes. On their way in, Dude asked Dan, "I hear your mama's coming home soon?"

Dan's face brightened. "Yep, she'll be home tonight! I can hardly wait." He smelled meat smoking when he walked into the barn, making his stomach grumble in hunger. It was the sausage hanging in the smoke house, reaching perfection for the Thanksgiving feast. It sure smelled better than the manure he would soon be shoveling.

The men walked over to the work bench and appeared to start fiddling with a small motor, but they were watching the boy and giving each other conspiratorial winks.

Dan leaned against a wall to take off his tennis shoes, then he pulled up the coveralls his Aunt Mary bought him from the thrift store. Once that was on and zipped up, he put on his work boots and waited for instructions.

On cue, Aunt Fara came walking out of the small room off the barn, known as "the office." Her pipe dangled from her lips. "Hey, you," she said, walking over casually and giving Dan's shoulder a squeeze. "How's work treatin' ya so far?" Her jacket smelled of tobacco, adding to the other wonderful aromas in the barn.

"So far so good, Aunt Fara," he said. She wasn't much taller than he was, so their gazes were nearly eye to eye. "I can't wait to start making real money. Allowances don't count as real money, ya know? Hey, when do I get paid anyway?" he asked boldly.

Chod and Dude turned around when the subject of payday came up, and Dan instantly regretted his question. They saw their recent lesson in pride flash across his little pea brain, and his face turned red as a beet, making both men smile with satisfaction.

Suddenly, Dan realized that what those men thought of him mattered. Right before he could back-pedal, Fara jumped in and saved him. "You'll get paid once a week, like everyone else 'round here, but you won't get paid unless you earn it, get it?"

"Got it," Dan said with big eyes, and meant it.

"What're you going to do with all that money anyway?" Fara asked, humoring the kid.

The boy jumped on that so fast one would've thought he'd been making a list. "First, I'm going to buy my mom some new clothes. She can't go around town in those orange things she's been wearing. Then, I'm going to take my mom and Aunt Mary to Big D's Steak house. Then, I'm going to save up for a dirt bike. Then, I might put some in the bank. Then I'm . . ."

Fara could tell that his list of wants was long, and could possibly go on forever, but daylight was a-burning, so she interrupted him, "Well, you're in luck, son, 'cause we're going to be short a hand here real soon and we'll be needing another good one. That means you'll have plenty of money to buy what you want. But right now, you're going to be cleaning out the office," Fara said, pointing. "It's one hell of a mess. When you're done in there you can go home, take a few days off for the holiday. But, after Thanksgiving, it's back to work. That sound okay to you?"

"Sounds good to me, Aunt Fara," he said, thinking about how he couldn't wait for the day to be over so he could get home and see his mom.

Fara and the men watched Dan walk across the room to the office door, wearing coveralls that bore someone else's name across the back, maneuvering around farm equipment and miscellaneous parts. They knew he was anticipating seeing a terrible mess inside the empty room, but they also knew something else.

Fara unconsciously grabbed hold of her two brothers' hands as Dan went for the doorknob, and when the squeal of surprise and delight came pouring out of that room, they knew it was time for them to go.

Before they'd made it to the exit they heard, "Mom, you're here! You're really here! Then, "Hey, where'd ya get those new clothes?"

ALMOST THANKSGIVING

Back at the Roberts' farm, Eileen and Katherine had just finished decorating the center of the tables with Eliza's donated harvest. Pumpkins, Indian corn, and an occasional gourd highlighted each of the beautiful wooden tables that stretched the length of the barn.

The posts were dressed in cornstalk bundles, and the simple bandstand was now defined by a circle of straw bales. The only thing left to do was disguise the plethora of card tables in white sheets where the food and drink would be placed.

For most of the morning, Betty sat next to the wood stove with her eyes glued to the stack of wood piled in front of her. Only once did she leave her warm, safe spot, shuffling over to the dwindling pile of corn near the calves' pen. Eileen didn't intervene, but she did stop what she was doing to monitor, just in case. The barn floor was uneven, and the old woman's shuffling put her at a greater risk of falling.

Eileen watched Betty bend down on one knee to feed Bob, and then Daisy, each an ear of corn, one at a time, through the slats in their pens. She was a natural. It was no secret that feeding and caring for the animals was once her favorite part of rural life, a passion she shared and passed on to her son, Charly.

Eileen briefly entertained the idea of getting more animals for Betty, as a type of medicine, but as soon as the thought entered her head, she saw that bewildered look return to Betty's face. Her eyes began to search the very same barn she'd spent most of her life in for something familiar. Seeing her bafflement was ugly and sad, all at the same time.

Dementia was not going to let her stay in this world or the old one. Like a hungry monster, it would not be satisfied until it gobbled her all up.

In the short time it took Eileen to walk over and lead Betty back to the warm seat by the stove, she was once again a shell of a woman, willing to be led anywhere by anyone.

Katherine had called it quits for the day and watched her daughter from one of the benches. She was proud of the woman her little girl had become but also terrified to witness the decline of the once sharp and vibrant Betty Lou.

After Betty was seated and safe, Eileen climbed a ladder near the stove and hung orange crepe paper along the rafters above, not taking notice of the two birds that hopped along the old timbers in front of her hands.

When she had finished, she folded the ladder and set it against a wall, she then sat down next to her mother to admire the colors surrounding them.

The barn and the tables looked incredible, better than you'd find in the Thanksgiving addition of Country Living. It was entirely ready for guests.

After a few minutes, Hugh and Bob came in, each carrying a bottle of Pabst Blue Ribbon. Katherine's eyes instantly zeroed in on the beers, and she mean-mugged her husband on his way to the table.

Once upon a time, Bob drank too much. For thirty-some-odd years Bob came home late most days, sloppy with alcohol, and often, foul words. Only to wake the next day without any consequences for his wife's unhappiness. She had threatened him with divorce on occasion but never made any moves in that direction.

Then one day, out of the blue, he just quit drinking, never admitting to anyone—including himself—that it had been a problem.

In truth, it was his age that motivated him, not his wife's repeated threats. Like many who crest that hill, he simply woke up one day and acknowledged that his life was almost over, and with deep clarity, decided to be a sober part of it.

Of course, Katherine was happy when he quit— actually, more relieved than happy. Sadly, though, by this point in their lives she had a whole lot of anger and resentment stored up, and it didn't just disappear with the drinking. It was something she consciously worked on because she loved the man.

Seeing her face, Bob instantly felt the need to defend himself. "Somethin' about a holiday makes a man feel like he's not on any schedule and can do whatever he wants to do. Isn't that right, Hugh?"

"That's right, buddy," Hugh said, stopping to take a drink from his bottle.

"Like you're ever on any schedule?" Katherine said, forcing a chuckle. "Just so you don't get tuned up, dear. I have lots of cooking to do tonight, and I need you to be sober enough to drive us home!"

"Not to worry, this isn't my first rodeo, nor is it my last," he added with sheepish smile, proud that he'd held his ground, even though it wasn't necessary.

"So, what do you think, guys?" Eileen asked, motioning around the room.

"It's beautiful," Hugh said, searching the room for Betty and finding her near the wood stove, eyes fixed on the stacked firewood. He thought she looked pale, but the lighting was spotty. It wasn't until he walked up right alongside her that he realized there was no question about her color; there was none.

The others sat talking while Hugh set his half empty bottle of beer down between a couple pieces of split wood. When he turned back around, he saw Boy standing on Betty's left shoulder.

Betty didn't look at Hugh. Nor did she acknowledge the bird that not long ago had been her Boy, their savior.

Hugh gently scooted the bird off her shoulder, realizing how he hadn't thought about it for a while, not since his wife's attention had switched over to the doll, which she no longer searched for either.

The bird flew above them and landed on the rafter next to another bird that looked just like him. Hugh was glad the little guy had found a friend, and glad that his wife, despite all her misery, had insisted on saving him. In turn, the bird had given them gifts that, in his mind, were nothing short of miracles.

Before tending to Betty, he gave thanks to the bird called Boy.

THE ASHLEY/MORGAN HOME

Leila, five foot three and weighing only one hundred and ten pounds stood next to her son who at ten years old was already closing in on her height. Her light brown hair shined, much like her face and almond eyes. She sipped her coffee and watched her son pour his cereal, taking in every move he made. He looked so much like his father that it tugged on her heart a bit, but not enough to take away from the happiness she felt for being with her family or the gratitude of her freedom.

Dan asked his mother to pick him up after school and drive him to Comanche for "just a minute." When she asked him why he wanted to go, he said, very matter-of-factly, "There's something I want to talk to dad about."

Leila was caught off guard, so she looked to her sister for a hint, anything that could assist with an answer.

Mary was busy at the table, gathering the papers she'd graded the night before and cramming them into her pack. She looked up and met her sister's eyes but didn't have any clues to offer. She merely shrugged her shoulders and smiled, deciding to take a backseat for the next few days and intervene only if it was really needed.

Mary knew that Leila still had the burden of telling Dan she would be leaving after Thanksgiving. Time was short between mother and son, so she was staying out of their business, as hard as it was for her to do. For once, she was relieved to be going to school.

It was as if Leila read her sister's mind. She turned back to her son, who waited for an answer. "How about this, honey? You don't go to school today, and we go wherever you want to go? That is, unless you want to go to school."

Dan automatically looked over to his aunt for permission. She was the rule-maker, the enforcer of everything in his life. She winked to let him know it was okay, feeling a little guilty that he looked to her for permission. Mary felt a tug on her heart. She loved him like he was her own; she couldn't help it. It's just what happened when you took care of a child and made them the priority in your life.

And like everything that involves love, heartache is part of what you sign up for, whether or not you know it at the time.

Mary knew the day would come when she'd have to let go of Dan. Even though her brain told her she was prepared for it, her heart was calling her head a liar.

"You think I'm crazy? Course I don't want to go to school. I want to spend the day with you, mom!" Dan looked over to his aunt again. "Thanks, Aunt Mary," he said.

"You're welcome." Mary chuckled. "I'll see you two this evening." Then she quickly disappeared through the doorway.

"If we leave right now, we can eat at that pancake house in Comanche. Remember the place with the huge pancakes and all the sausage gravy a person could ever want?" Dan asked excitedly.

"Of course, I remember it. Annie's was our favorite spot. Sure baby, that sounds good. And after you've talked to your dad, maybe you and I can talk for a while."

"I'm so glad you're home, mom," Dan said, hugging his mother. "I'm so glad you're home!"

Clearing the lump in her throat, she whispered, "Me too, now let's go see if that car of ours will start."

SARAH'S STABLES

Over at Sarah's, the pecan pies were all baked and cooling on the porch, set up high enough that her two dogs, or any other critters, couldn't help themselves to a treat. At least she hoped they couldn't.

She'd already shot two squirrels that had looked at the porch suspiciously, and though she really didn't want to shoot any more of them, she would protect the pies she'd spent all morning making.

Sarah leaned her .22 rifle against the house and stepped down from the porch. She needed to get Johnny, one of her favorite horses, saddled and ready to ride. She didn't have any lessons today, but she did have a guest coming out.

Austen would soon be arriving with his own horse and trailer. The day before they'd decided to take a long ride down gravel roads, just to see how their horses would do together. If everything went as planned, they'd ride the back roads to the Roberts' farm the following day for Thanksgiving.

On her way to the stable, she stuck out her tongue, licking random snowflakes from the air and thinking as she did how the new falling snow made everything more romantic. Her anticipation over her handsome guest's arrival made her feel more alive than she'd ever felt before.

If their test ride was a success, which Sarah was certain it would be, they would take her pies, along with whatever wild rice concoction Austen made, to the Roberts' in his truck later that evening. That way, they wouldn't have to worry about the impossible task of packing their food by horseback the next day.

She was excited for many reasons, but most of all she was thrilled to be the "pilgrim" this particular Indian chose to be with for Thanksgiving.

HEINS' HOG FARM

Mike and Evert Heins' smoke house had been filled to capacity for the past two days, overflowing with young turkeys and hams; raised and butchered by the Heins themselves.

The smoke that filled the air was blinding, like a fog that wouldn't lift. It wafted over the dead grass, frozen limp, and drooping, as if the fields were weeping. Those lucky enough to be outside could catch a whiff of Thanksgiving on the breeze.

The inside of the house held wonderful smells of its own, thanks to Mike's wife, Debra. Her oyster stuffing was to die for. She once owned her own restaurant and followed her instincts to call Eileen and let her know that it was full of fresh oysters. If someone at the feast had a shellfish allergy, she didn't want anyone to literally die from eating her stuffing.

Food allergies were something you never thought about in the old days. You just ate what was served and found out later if it made you sick. But times change.

Evert's wife, Barbara, had been gone five years now, and if it hadn't been for his son and daughter-in-law, he would've given up on holidays all together.

Pastor Dale told him a few years back, while trying to talk him into spending Thanksgiving with him and his wife, Linda Rae, that family are those you surround yourself with "whether or not they're blood."

It wasn't until this moment, as he removed the meat from the smoker and transferred it into the large cooler in his barn, that he understood what his pastor meant.

In his heart, he'd always known that people he called friends were a part of him, close enough to consider family. He was excited for the next day, eager to be able to share his bounty with the people he cared for and loved.

THE GRAHAM HOME

Patty and Leroy worked together in their kitchen, baking a variety of casseroles with the sweet yams and green beans from their garden they'd canned only a few months before. They were proud to share their season of hard work with the gathering at the Roberts' farm, and equally proud to be included.

Leroy pinched Patty on her plump rump as she bent over to open the oven door. Her giggle was infectious, and soon they both were laughing. Laughter had always been their strong point. It was part of what kept their thirty-some-odd years together so very "together."

The only things they argued about were Patty's smoking and Leroy's nail biting. She hated with a passion how Leroy bit his nails down to the quick, and he hated her addiction to cigarettes. Neither issue was earth-shattering, but the two would repeat the same arguments a hundred times before they died, because those were the only things, they disliked about each other.

Leroy was built like a bull and had a bush of curly black hair turned salt and pepper which he always stuffed under a cap of some kind. He retired from logging after watching his best friend get crushed to death by a skidder. He lost his wife to cancer that same year. That year would have changed him forever, and not in a good way, until he saw Patty in the parking lot of the post office one summer's day. She'd dropped her mail, scattering it all over the lot, just as Leroy pulled in after his first day of work as a mail carrier. It was a job he'd taken only because he was bored, a reason to get out of the house—which he'd needed.

Seeing her scrambling to retrieve her mail, he thought she was just the right size for a woman. Leroy liked meat on a woman's bones. Skinny women always reminded him of something out of National Geographic—a starving tribe member of one kind or another.

He parked his vehicle, then went over and bent down to help her pick up the envelopes blowing around the lot. But Leroy had done more than grab mail off the ground; he'd also peeked down Patty's shirt at her breasts. He hadn't meant to be rude, or seem like a pig, but those two large breasts dangled in front of him like a pair of playful devils, waving at him.

Suddenly, Leroy could feel her eyes boring into him. He'd been caught, and because he really wasn't a pig of a man, and rather shy, he was acutely embarrassed and felt the need to apologize—not for being a creep, but for being human. His tongue stuck in his throat when he raised his head and looked into the eyes of the most beautiful woman he'd ever seen. Those breasts were something, all right, but they were nothing compared to her face.

It was as if a spell had been cast in the post office parking lot that day. Two lonely people who thought their destiny was to be alone for the rest of their lives found each other.

Patty had never had a boyfriend. She always believed and accepted that no one would ever want her. She'd been self-conscious about her weight since childhood, due in part to her father's constant harsh remarks about her size. He called her "chubby checkers" and "fat ass," and not just in private either. He said that fat people were lazy, and for years she fantasized about standing up to him, especially about the lazy part, because it was her mother who supported the family, not him. Her dad sat on the couch all day, watching TV in his underwear, while her mother worked like a dog at the bread factory in town, coming home to make dinner for him before even sitting down.

To say that his daughter resented him would be an understatement.

Patty wore her inferiority complex into adulthood. Thanks to dear old dad it was always present and grew uglier with age, like a faded tattoo. She cried a lot back then, but not on the day her father died. Neither did her mother cry. Instead, they went to Red Lobster and celebrated their freedom.

"Hey honey," her husband began as they worked on the casseroles. "How 'bout when we're done in here, we treat ourselves and go to town for dinner? Maybe even have a drink or three. Then, when we come home, we can play cops and robbers. I'll be the cop and you be the robber."

Patty broke out in more laughter, but managed to squeak out, "Oh, I like being the bad one!"

CHARLES & ELIZA (SNOOPY PANTS) REEVE

Charles Reeve was busy unloading the wine from his truck to Eliza's car. It was cheap carton wine, bought at Sam's Club, but they weren't connoisseurs, and they hoped the guests at the Roberts' farm weren't either. The Reeves weren't cheap. They were frugal and proud of the way being careful with money had paid off in their lives.

Both of them had always worked, they just never made a lot of money doing it. It was only because they'd been bean counters that they had a home that was paid for and were comfortable in their retirement.

They'd both grown up poor, and when you grow up that way you either learn how to be careful with money, or you spend it faster than you can make it. There's not a lot of in between. It's sort of like growing up around an alcoholic. Either you swear off drinking, or you drink like a fish.

Not having grown up on farms, like many of their friends had, meant that when the money ran out, so did the food. When times were tough on a farm, the families might not have had much, but come mealtime, there was always food on the table.

Other than being short and round, being hungry as kids was one of the few things Charles and Eliza had in common, and something neither of them would ever forget, nor wish on another living soul.

They'd pinched and saved for years so that their children could go to college. College wasn't an option in their household, but a requirement. They didn't want their children to struggle through life as they had. The Reeves believed that a college education was the ticket out of poverty—and they were right. All three of their children were professionals of one kind or another. That was the Reeves' single biggest accomplishment in life.

Charles still chose to work part-time delivering pizzas on the weekends, but that wasn't because they needed the extra money as much as it was a chance for Charles to get out of the house and have space from his wife.

There was no question that they cared for one another, but they were as different as peas and carrots— compatible, but not alike. After fifty years together, and with divorce not an option, they'd learned how to make their marriage work and to appreciate each other. Having space, as they called it, worked for them.

While Charles was outside, Eliza sat in their living room with her feet up on a chair. Her ankles were swollen, a common occurrence nowadays. Not only was she overweight, but her volunteer schedule kept her on her feet far longer than any human being should be. But you couldn't tell her that. Eliza believed that the way to heaven was through good deeds, and if there truly was such a place as heaven, she most certainly deserved to be first in line. Her heart was as big as her ankles, if not bigger.

THE HAMILTONS

The Hamilton's were an ambitious young family with jobs that sucked more than forty hours a week out of them. Tom was the head pharmacist at Walgreen's in Ottumwa, and Tennille was the manager of the largest grain mill in the county. Their ten-year-old twins, Jason and Kary Lynn, also had schedules nearly as time consuming as their parents.

By the time they all got home, there was often no time for home-cooked meals, so Tennille would stop somewhere along her way and pick up a meal that someone else had made.

The American dream of his and her SUV's, watching sports, lavish vacations, and a house that was too big for one person to clean cost their family a lot more than money.

With Thanksgiving a few hours away, Tennille felt stressed. The band was their contribution to the Roberts' festivities, and though that was welcomed by all who would attend, it just wasn't enough for Tennille. She had been raised in a household where home-cooked meals were as natural as having two parents living together. It felt odd to not be making something yummy for

Thanksgiving, because that wasn't the way she was raised. Cooking used to be the buildup to a big day; it was what made a holiday feel like a holiday. She longed for the good old days, feeling guilty and disappointed in herself for allowing her busy life to get in the way of tradition.

On her way home, Tennille stopped at the Canteen Lunch under the interstate bridge and purchased their famous loose meat sandwiches and fries. Inhaling the food as she drove the ten miles home, she promised herself that her priorities were going to change.

Tom was also on his way home, but first he had to pick up the kids from their swimming lessons at the Y. Usually, his drive home gave him time to unwind, but this evening was different. He felt unnerved as he thought about his wife and his kids. He suddenly realized that he missed them even though they were living under the same roof. He knew he and his wife were growing apart, not because they were short on love, but because they were short on time. He decided that it was no longer acceptable.

His kids seemed unfazed by the lack of time they spent together, but out of fairness, how could someone miss something they haven't had? That question filled him with shame as he pulled into the lot at the Y and saw both of his children standing on the sidewalk, glued to their cell phones.

"Stuff!" he grumbled out loud. All the stuff in the world simply couldn't replace what they were missing: each other. Tom sat in his car and watched his kids' little fingers move like lightning across the screens of their phones, wondering just how long it would take for them to look up and see him sitting there. The shame he'd felt quickly morphed into annoyance. He honked the horn once, then kept his hand pressed on it to embarrass them.

Embarrassment, if created without intent to harm, made a kid tough, he reasoned. He remembered back to when he was a teenager and "too cool" to be seen with his parents, but his mother insisted that he go everywhere with them anyway. The minute his parents cleared the door of whatever store they dragged him into, he would go in the opposite direction, pretending to anyone who might give a damn that he was alone and definitely *not* with his parents.

Even though Tom couldn't have imagined it, his mother had once been a teenager herself, and she handled his embarrassment by embarrassing him even more. She would stand in the middle of an aisle and holler his name until she'd flushed him out of hiding, his hesitant appearance meant just to shut her up. He was embarrassed alright, but her tactic toughened him up enough that he eventually quit working so hard at being cool.

His children both looked up in horror from their phones. Kary Lynn held up her arms and mouthed, "Enough, already!"

When they jumped in the car, and before they could tell him what a dork he was, he said, "Guess what we're NOT taking with us to Thanksgiving?"

MARY AND CHOD

Mary arrived home from school the evening before Thanksgiving and set about boiling water for the Jell-O desserts she was making for the feast. After filling the kettle, she sat down to pull off the shoes that were killing her feet, when she heard a knock at the door. She kicked her shoes to the side of the hallway where they hit the wall with a couple of loud thuds.

Opening the door, she was surprised to find Chod standing there.

"Hey, can I come in?" he asked through the screen door.

She shrugged her shoulders, but quickly tried to pretend that she hadn't, and opened the door wide enough for the huge man to pass through.

"Of course, is everything all right?"

The last time Mary had seen Chod was when he picked up her nephew at school to work at Fara's. She felt the same tug on her heart that day that she felt now.

"You wouldn't happen to have any coffee made, would you?" Chod asked, standing in the narrow hallway, way too close to her for comfort.

"I don't, but I can make some. Come on in and take a seat, it'll only take me a minute." The task of making coffee momentarily saved her. She damn near ran from the hallway and the unbearable closeness of this gentle giant.

Chod followed her into the kitchen and took a seat at the table. Mary could feel his eyes on her back. Without turning around, she asked, "So what's up?"

When he didn't answer, she was forced to face him again. He sat at her table with tears in his eyes, trying with everything he had to speak.

"Mary," he finally got out, "I know about your cancer. It's no secret, and of course I know about Leila having to go away again." Clearing his throat, he looked straight at her. "I want you to know that I care. I have never stopped caring about you." He paused to wipe his eyes, then blow his nose with the handkerchief he'd pulled out of his back pocket.

Mary didn't know what to say, but she opened her mouth anyway, prepared to banish the awkwardness that hung in the air. Before she could speak, he stood up and closed the distance between them.

She backed up as far as she could, until her calves were pressed against the lower cabinets. She even leaned back against the counter, but he kept on coming. He was only inches away from her, forcing her to look up into his face or be smothered in the chest she'd so desperately missed.

"Mary, I came here today to tell you something, and I'm not leaving until I do. I want to help you and I want you to let me help you." Seeing the pain in her face, he continued while he still had the stones. "I love you, Mary, and even if you don't love me anymore, I want to help you. Please!" Then, just like that, he turned around and retreated to the chair at the table, as if what he'd just said took every ounce of his energy and he had to sit down or fall down.

She watched his large frame collapse into the chair. Mary felt like the wind had just been knocked out of her, but finally she opened her mouth again. This time words came out. "Chod, you sweet man, I never stopped loving you. The only reason I stopped seeing you was because my life changed. I promised my sister I would take care of Dan, remember? I thought you understood that."

He nodded. "I did understand, and I still do understand, but right now you don't have to take care of anybody but you, and I want to be with you as you go through this. The question is, will you let me?"

"What about Dan? And what about your work at the ranch?" she asked.

Now it was Mary closing the distance between them, standing right in front of the seated giant.

"My sister and brother will make sure Dan's okay, you know that", he said. "And the ranch won't miss me much. I figure I can spend the week with you in Des Moines, and after your chemo treatments we'll drive back home for the weekends. That way you can see Dan, and I can catch up on my work."

The coffee maker hissed as it finished brewing, but they no longer cared about coffee. Mary eased her way in between his legs, then cradled his balding head in her hands. She kissed the top of it before guiding it onto her chest.

"I was afraid you thought I had too many miles on me," he admitted, mumbling into her blouse.

"Never," she whispered.

The screen door opened, then slammed shut. Chod's head snapped up and out of its cradle at lightning speed, but there was no time to stand up and pretend that there was no more than just coffee brewing in that kitchen.

Mary froze, her face turning a shade you wouldn't find on any color chart as Leila walked into the kitchen. Dan's mom took in the scene at the table, a large grin spreading across her face. "Hi Chod," she said. "Long time no see."

Before Chod could return the greeting, he heard Dan come barreling down the hallway, stopping in the kitchen doorway to see what everyone was up to. He knew Chod was there because he'd seen his truck parked out front. Since he just had the conversation with his mom about his living and working at the Kremer Ranch for a few months, he assumed Chod's visit was all business. It took the poor kid a few seconds before he caught onto the fact that his aunt was holding his new employer's head in both hands, just a bit too close to her breasts.

When he did get the picture, everyone in the room watched as his mouth fell open, magnifying the empty whole where a tooth had once lived. The scene in the kitchen was quickly becoming comical. So much so that the adults were working hard at suppressing their laughter.

Dan looked at his aunt and then to Chod. Then he slowly shut his mouth and walked in closer, trying to assess exactly what was happening. "Chod?" he blurted out. "Are you all right, sir?"

Chod nodded as a laugh escaped Leila's mouth.

Dan then looked at his aunt, his blonde hair falling over his accusing eyes and his mouth twisting in disgust. "Aunt Mary! What the heck are you doing to my boss?"

Mary could no longer contain herself. She cracked up.

Soon, everyone in the kitchen—including Dan—was laughing from somewhere deep down in their bellies, filling the small space with something long overdue and as essential as marrow to bone.

PASTOR DALE & LINDA RAE

Pastor Dale had just finished his Wednesday confirmation class. The simple stone church was empty and quiet as he began stacking the chairs against the wall while his wife, Linda, tidied up the room.

Both were eager to get home and start breading and frying a ridiculous amount of chicken livers, after which Linda was going to duplicate her grandmother's butter rolls for the feast. It would be a late night in the kitchen, but an expected one this time of year.

Quietly, they anticipated the warmth and familiarity of the holidays as they tackled the tasks ahead.

Linda worked as fast as her diseased body would allow. Her MS was claiming more and more ownership of her limbs, leaving her with a numbness and an annoying fatigue, neither of which stopped her from being a part of whatever was going on.

Dale watched her work from across the room, remembering the day he'd first laid eyes on her. He thought at the time that she looked like the woman who played Wonder Woman in the TV series. In truth, she did— voluminous jet-black hair, sparkling blue eyes, cherry lips—just without the outfit.

Watching her work now, with only one side of her body functioning, he decided she was indeed Wonder Woman. His wife never complained about what was happening to her mind and body. She believed her suffering was God's will. She trusted with all her heart and soul that she was chosen by Him to endure it, and for that reason alone she never complained.

Dale knew his wife was stronger than he was when it came to selflessness. He admitted to her from time to time that he was angry with God, even as he watched her calmly accept transforming into a shadow of what she'd once been.

Linda knew each scripture upside down and inside out, quoting appropriate ones whenever her husband needed to be pulled from the darkness of fear for her. She always had a way of making things make sense to him. It was a gift she had, one that had saved him so many years before.

In his late twenties, suffering from clinical depression, Dale lost his job and, with no family to turn to for help, he soon lost his apartment as well. Homeless and penniless, he ended up in a shelter, one where Linda was teaching Bible studies twice a week.

He became interested in her teachings, and after a few short months, he was committed to God. Three years later, he became pastor of his own church and husband to his very own "Wonder Woman."

Dale walked over to his wife and gently took her arm as she wiped the last table. "It's time we go home," he said. "You need to take a break before we dive into all that cooking. I'll run you a bath, and while you're soaking, I'll make us something good to eat. How's that sound, sweetie?"

Taking his offered arm, she said, "Sounds great, I'm pooped."

They were locking up the back door to the church when the sound of footsteps came from behind them. They found a wiry old man standing on the sidewalk, a duffel bag in one hand and a cigarette in the other. He was so thin it looked like a strong wind could blow him down the street.

"Pastor Dale?" the man asked.

Dale nodded, his muscles stiffening slightly.

"I hear you're The Man." He looked over at Linda and nodded again. "And I hear you're The Man too," he said with a toothless smile.

Dale moved protectively between his wife and the stranger, asking, "What can we do for you, sir?"

"Name's Allen, Allen Archer. I was told that you were the one to see if I needed help, and right now I'm in need of help."

A layer of tenderness warmed Dale's voice. "What kind of help are you looking for?"

"I'm waiting for a bed to open up at a treatment center in Des Moines. They say I can't get in until the Friday after Thanksgiving. I was hoping you could help me find a place to stay for the next two nights, and maybe lend me a couple bucks for something to eat."

"Archer?" Dale said. "I knew a guy named Archer once, a quarterback. I played football with him at ISU. You any relation?"

The man hung his head. "Once upon a time that was me, Dale. Don't blame you for not recognizing me. Once my dad died, I got caught up in some bad stuff. Spent all my money on drugs, even the money he left me. Lost my job, my wife, and then my kids. Now here I am, alone and back in Ottumwa trying to pick up the pieces before there aren't any left to pick up."

The man's cigarette fell from his stained fingers, landing on the ground along with his duffel bag. He started to cry into his dirty hands like a baby.

Dale walked over to the man he'd once known. He placed a hand on the bony shoulder and said compassionately, "You're not alone Allen. Jesus is your friend."

Allen removed his hands from his face. "The only friend I've had up until recently goes by the name of meth and believe me when I say I'm ready for a different one."

"I believe you, Allen," Dale said, unlocking the door. "How about you and I take a ride. I have a good friend who runs a shelter out of an old farm in Eldon called the Red Rooster Inn. He'll be happy to feed you and give you a bed for a couple nights. Then when the treatment center's ready for you, I'll drive you there myself."

Before Allen could say anything, Linda added, "How about you go with Dale and get settled in, then we'll pick you up in the morning and you can spend Thanksgiving with us and some of our friends. There'll be plenty of food and, trust me, they won't mind."

"Sounds too good to be true." Allen twisted his upper lip into a smile and smoothed his shaggy hair over his forehead. Then, in a poor attempt at an Elvis impersonation, he said, "Thank you. Thank you very much!" Bad as it was, it made Dale grin. He was more than happy to help Allen. At the same time, he no longer really knew him, much less trusted him, so he turned around and walked his wife back into the church to wait for his return.

When they'd cleared the doors, she smiled and squeezed his hand. "This is going to be the best Thanksgiving ever."

"Dang tootin'," he agreed with a wink.

Boy and Girl

Boy and his female double were playing in the Roberts'
fields, dodging each other and the snowflakes gently falling
from the sky.

They played until they grew hungry and needed a break,
which they took in the ancient oak tree on the levy near the
river. After a few minutes of rest, Boy's friend took flight again,
flitting from one rotten tree to another. She finally settled on
one near the fence line, drilling relentlessly into its hollow core.

Her beak was stuffed with food when she landed back on
the branch next to Boy. She leaned close to him, offering what
she'd just worked so hard to gather, and he gobbled it right up.

As grateful as he was for the flies and abundance of
sunflower seeds he'd been eating for the past few weeks, he had
to admit that this meal was much more satisfying.

Pleased that he was pleased, the female bird left the branch
to go get more.

Boy felt embarrassed for not having the skills to find his
own food. Apparently, hitting the window had cost him more
than his ability to fly. Although his body was now strong, his
memory was going to take a little more time to return.

Just as she arrived back at the tree with more food, a
massive flock of birds flew over them in a synchronized pattern,

landing on the barren field just long enough to get the energy to do it again and again.

As they ate and watched the show, Boy could hardly believe his eyes. There were so many birds out there, and all of them looked like him.

His new lady love nestled in close, and when he turned to look into her big black eyes, he saw longing he couldn't ignore, lighting a flame in him that he never thought possible.

Finally, he knew what he must do.

He left the tree and flew across the field and pasture, passing the lounging Bob and Daisy, on his way to the house with the faded shutters.

He circled the chicken coop; the fearless rooster the only one outside, not bothered by the falling snow. Then, with no competition in sight, the large fowl pecked at the ground feverishly, looking up to acknowledge Boy as he passed over before returning to his pecking.

Boy's heart pounded with excitement. "I am Boy," he sang at the top of his lungs.

Far off in the old oak tree came a faint return. "I know who you are, Boy, and when you return to me, I will teach you what you are."

Boy landed on the rotten windowsill—inches from the pane of glass that had nearly cost him his life—and prepared to say goodbye. But when he looked through the glass his little heart sank.

Something was wrong. He could feel it. As he shook off the snow that was quickly coating his body, he knew he couldn't leave, not now. And he knew the others wouldn't wait long for him. So be it, he told himself. If he were lucky, he would find them again in the spring.

A THANKSGIVING MIRACLE

Since Eileen's plans were to spend the entire day inside baking, she offered to watch Betty so that Hugh could be free to do as he pleased. She had no problem giving her mother-in-law a bath. She'd been giving her one on a regular basis for some time. Nor did she mind babysitting her, but this time Hugh had resisted, saying he didn't want to go out today. The truth was that he didn't want to leave his wife's side.

"Something isn't right," he told Eileen. "You don't spend most of your life with someone and not know these things."

So, all morning he sat on the couch next to Betty's chair, making several unsuccessful attempts to read while she slept. The only time he'd left the couch was to go to the bathroom and let a meowing Mrs. Nickels out.

He caught Eileen peeking in at him a time or two from the kitchen where she was busy making and baking half a dozen pineapple upside-down cakes.

The house smelled like a home, and he was grateful for that, more than he could ever say. If it weren't for his concern for Betty, Eileen knew he'd be soaking up the feeling of Thanksgiving as she was.

She knew this because he was hungry for it, and it showed in everything he'd been doing up to this point. But today he was too preoccupied, watching his wife's chest rise and fall, sitting on the edge of the couch ready to jump up at any moment.

Eileen worried because he worried. "Something you want to talk about, Hugh?" she asked from the kitchen as she removed two golden cakes from the oven and set them on the counter to cool. She bent down and opened the oven door to put the last of the waiting pans in, hearing no answer from the other room. She went towards the counter that bordered the living room, peering over to see if Hugh and Betty were still there.

They were, but Hugh was no longer on the edge of the couch. He was on the floor, kneeling in front of the chair that held a limp body. Betty's head hung to one side like a rag doll. Her small mouth was open enough to see her tongue, hanging half in and half out. Hugh's head lay in her lap, his large body convulsing silently with pain.

"Oh my God," Eileen cried, taking it all in and running to them. She got down on the floor behind Hugh and put her arms as far around him as she could. Her left hand reached up for the tiny wrist that dangled over the arm of the chair. There was no pulse. Betty was gone, but this time she wouldn't be found in the yard or the chicken coop. She was *gone*, gone.

"I'm so sorry, Hugh. So, so sorry," she whispered into the back of his flannel shirt.

They stayed that way for a few minutes before he lifted his head. "Did you know that in her day, Betty was a hell of a dancer?"

Eileen shook her head, even though she did know. She let him ramble.

"She was one hell of dancer, best dance partner I ever had. I guess she was the only dance partner I ever had," he mumbled, a small laugh escaping as the tears ran down his face.

"I know it sounds selfish, but I was really looking forward to Thanksgiving so we could dance again. Just one more dance. Damn it!" He lay his head back down and sobbed some more.

It wasn't selfish at all, and as much as Eileen wanted to tell him that, she kept quiet. This was his time. Even so, she wasn't going to leave him alone. Not now, not ever.

Eileen rested her head on his large back and listened to his sobs, feeling more helpless than she'd felt in her entire life. After a while, she felt a tug on her hair. It was snagged or caught somewhere on Hugh's shirt. She lifted her head after feeling a particularly hard pull.

"Holy shit!" Eileen gasped, falling backwards onto the floor and startling Hugh. He lifted his head and looked back at her, but all she could do was point.

Hugh's eyes followed her finger back to the chair. He too gasped when he saw a wide-eyed Betty starring back, holding a tuft of Eileen's hair in her hand.

Hugh jumped up off the floor and bent over to hold his no longer dead wife. However, Betty would have none of it. She slapped her stunned husband away like a bothersome fly.

"She's back!" he said, breathlessly straightening his old body. "By God, she's back!"

Eileen stayed put on the floor, frozen stiff with shock. She'd heard of people waking up from a coma, but not death. Never ever had she heard of anyone coming back from the dead, not in real life anyway. Could this be real?

The utter quiet that fell over the room was so profound that you could hear the old house creak. At last, Hugh offered his hand to Eileen and helped her to her feet. They stood facing each other, both still in total disbelief, when the timer on the stove sounded, breaking the spell.

Before reaching the kitchen counter, Eileen turned back to look at Hugh and the now animated Betty, just to make sure she hadn't imagined the whole thing.

With a new urgency, she removed the cakes from the oven, then hurried back to the living room where Hugh once again sat on the couch. His hands formed a steeple while his eyes looked up to the stained ceiling above. His lips moved, but no sound came out.

Betty sat unaware in her chair by the window, just as she usually did, contentedly watching the snow fall outside.

When Eileen's gaze moved from Hugh to Betty, she saw the old woman smile at her own reflection in the glass. Beyond the window, Eileen caught the briefest glimpse of a bird as it lifted into the snowy afternoon and flew away.

"Hugh, don't you think we should take Betty to the hospital, just to get her checked out?" Eileen thought that she herself might need to be checked out too.

"No honey, I don't," he replied. "Whatever is going to happen to this woman is going to happen to her right here in her own house and on her own farm." Hugh glanced over to Wife, then added, smiling, "Besides, I believe the Lord has already checked her out."

Eileen didn't know what to say, so she walked over to him and placed a hand on his face where his tears had already dried. She was so thankful that Jacob was at school. Nothing she had seen just now could be explained, not in a million years. She thought whoever said that a parent has the answer to everything was just, well, full of shit.

Like a robot, she walked into the kitchen, opened the cabinet above the sink—the one that held the brandy—and poured herself a shot. As she raised the glass to her lips, she glanced out the window in time to see a swarm of birds flying by. As if on cue, they reversed direction, landing on the ground just outside.

Numb with shock and wonder, Eileen watched a single bird leave the group and fly over to the window, hovering in the air right in front of her. The tiny bird was so close that if the windowpane hadn't separated them, she could have reached out and touched it.

Bird and woman locked eyes, then the former jetted away, returning to the others who seemed to be waiting. Then they disappeared, as if they'd never been there at all.

With a shaky hand, Eileen again took down the bottle of brandy, this time filling the glass to the brim. Warm tears ran down her cheeks as she downed the liquor like the pro she wasn't.

Once the choking and gagging subsided, Eileen caught her breath and leaned against the sink, thinking about how there was no way in hell she would ever forget what just happened. With hesitation, she raised her head to look out the window, uncertain of what might await her on the other side.

Her heart smiled when she saw Jacob skipping up the gravel driveway towards the house, wearing a paper hat shaped like a turkey. Her thoughts turned to the big day ahead and to her gratitude for the gift of life and even death. The good, the bad, and the ugly—the numb nuts and the dick weeds—she was thankful for all of it.

She whispered to no one in particular, or possibly to everyone and everything, "Thanksgiving, here we come!"

About the Author

Anna Hamilton lives in Grand Marais Minnesota where she and her sister Sarah have over the past 28 years, owned and operated a number of restaurants along the Gunflint Trail and Grand Marais. The businesses have given them a platform to mentor those who need work ethics and life skills. In 2020 they created a non -profit called 'Hamilton Habitat'. A charitable organization that builds "affordable homes" for the working folks who normally would be pushed out of a popular tourist community.

Hamiltonhabitat.wordpress.com

'Boy' was created after Anna lost her father to Dementia. Her experience of being 'present' with her father during his illness changed her outlook on life and on death and the 'rules' for both "For the first time in my life I felt I had permission to lie to my dad. Anything that brought him comfort is what came out of my mouth. Just when sadness threatened to eat me alive is when, accidentally, I found joy. It was through the people I met, others who no longer knew who or where they were that made me laugh and cry and appreciate the journey I was on. Hope is what I found. That is what I wish for all who are touched by this disease.

"Once upon a time, this community saved me. I will give back to it what it has given to me, which is a chance to do better and a wonderful place to do it."

Thank you, Anna

CPSIA information can be obtained
at www.ICGtesting.com
Printed in the USA
FSHW020725080521
81246FS

9 781950 502400